Introduction to Social Security

Social security is a major part of government policy and social expenditure; we are all contributors to its funding via general taxation and social insurance, and we all receive benefits at some point in our lives. Against a background of recent controversies about the government's various proposals on social security reform and changes in the DSS ministerial team, *Introduction to Social Security* succeeds in consolidating, evaluating and presenting some of the most recent findings and thinking in the field of social security.

With chapters by leading contributors in their fields, this book covers such issues as: poverty, aims and development of social security, pensions policy, claiming entitlements, disability, 'race', women, and poverty in a European context. *Introduction to Social Security* is essential reading for students of social administration, social and public policy.

John Ditch is Professor of Social Policy at the University of York.

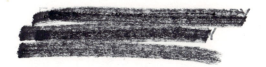

Introduction to Social Security

Policies, benefits and poverty

Edited by John Ditch

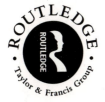

London and New York

First published 1999
by Routledge
11 New Fetter Lane, London EC4P 4EE

Simultaneously published in the USA and Canada
by Routledge
29 West 35th Street, New York, NY 10001

Routledge is an imprint of the Taylor & Francis Group

Typeset in Bembo by Routledge
Printed and bound in Great Britain by Clays Ltd, St Ives plc

British Library Cataloguing in Publication Data
A catalogue record for this book is available from the British
Library

Library of Congress Cataloging in Publication Data
Introduction to social security: policies, benefits, and poverty/
edited by John Ditch
p. cm.
Includes bibliographical references and index.
1. Social security – Great Britain. I. Ditch, John.
HD7165.I58 1999
368.4´00941–dc2199-26250
CIP

ISBN 0–415–21430–0 (hbk)
ISBN 0–415–21431–9 (pbk)

For Zoë Maria

Contents

x   Contents

Illustrations

Tables

Figures

Contributors

Pete Alcock is Professor of Social Policy in the Department of Social Policy at the University of Birmingham.

Sally Baldwin is Professor of Social Policy and Director of the Social Policy Research Unit at the University of York.

Helen Barnes is a Lecturer in the Department of Social Policy at the University of North London.

Jonathan Bradshaw is Professor of Social Policy in the Department of Social Policy and Social Work at the University of York.

Anne Corden is a Research Fellow in the Social Policy Research Unit at the University of York.

Gary Craig is a Professor of Social Policy in the School of Policy Studies at the University of Humberside.

John Ditch is Professor of Social Policy in the Department of Social Policy and Social Work at the University of York.

Eileen Evason is Professor of Social Policy in the Department of Social Policy at the University of Ulster

Eithne McLaughlin is Professor of Social Policy in the Department of Sociology & Social Policy at Queens University, Belfast.

Roy Sainsbury is a Senior Research Fellow in the Social Policy Research Unit at the University of York.

John Veit-Wilson is Professor of Social Policy in the Department of Social Policy at the University of Newcastle upon Tyne.

Preface

The development, management and delivery social security policy are central to any government's agenda: in the United Kingdom about £100 billion is spent annually, over 75,000 are employed in the Department of Social Security (and its constituent agencies) and no less than 25 million benefit recipients demand that it could and should not be otherwise. As if to match this commitment, the study of social security has long been at the heart of social policy as an academic subject. Indeed, research and teaching in the field of social security have become a minor industry. Every year the Department of Social Security commissions a substantial programme of research worth approximately £3.5 million, much of it conducted by specialists found in a small number of predominantly English universities. The resulting reports feed directly into the policy process, and after an exhaustive process of consultation and validation, are published to become part of the evidential base about the functioning of social security in the United Kingdom. There is now a substantial library of research findings, augmented by other dedicated studies into the strengths, weaknesses and possibilities for social security. Some of this material finds its way into teaching and training programmes and some gets re-cycled in literature reviews which are *de rigueur* in succeeding studies. But, somewhat surprisingly, much of this material remains known only to the professionals and *cogniscenti*. Indeed, it is remarkable that there are not more generalist texts, seeking to introduce social security to a wider policy and academic audience. This book attempts to bridge that gap: it provides a review of social security policy and practice which is informed by recent research but accessible to the non-specialist.

That this book appears at all is, however, a triumph of hope over experience and very much a tribute to those contributors who have remained loyal to the project. Each author has my sincere thanks for their fortitude as well as their scholarship. In the sands of North Africa it is said that caravans move at the speed of the slowest camel: we have lost a number of camels along the way and others have needed rather more water (and such like fluids) than was anticipated! But in addition to my splendid co-authors I must also thank Rebecca Harrison and Nathalie Constantino who word-processed the manuscript through its various iterations and thereby helped maintain my sense of purpose and equilibrium. Finally, I should like to thank Heather Gibson of Routledge who was both encouraging and supportive at just the right moment.

John Ditch
York
June 1999

Abbreviations

AA   Attendance Allowance
CAB   Citizens' Advice Bureau
CHAC   Central Housing Advisory Committee
CPAG   Child Poverty Action Group
CSA   Child Support Agency
DFEE   Department for Education and Employment
DHSS   Department of Health and Social Security
DIG   Disablement Income Group
DLA   Disability Living Allowance
DSS   Department of Social Security
DTER   Department for Transport, Environment and the Regions
DWA   Disability Working Allowance
ECPCP   European Community Programme to Combat Poverty
ESRC   Economic and Social Research Council
FC   Family Credit
FES   Family Expenditure Survey
FIS   Family Income Supplement
FRS   Family Resources Survey
HBAI   Households Below Average Income
HNIC   Housewives Non-Contributory Pension
ICA   Invalid Care Allowance
ILF   Independent Living Fund
IS   Income Support
JRF   Joseph Rowntree Foundation
LIS   Low Income Statistics
LSE   London School of Economics
MIS   Minimum Income Standards
NACAB   National Association of Citizens' Advice Bureaux
NCIP   Non-contributory Invalidity Pension
NIC   National Insurance Contribution

NIO   Northern Ireland Office
OPCS   Office of Population Censuses and Surveys
RPI   Retail Price Index
SBC   Supplementary Benefits Commission
SDA   Severe Disablement Allowance
SERPS   State Earnings-Related Pensions Scheme
UA   Unemployment Assistance

Introduction

Policies and current issues

John Ditch

There is a significant irony to be found at the heart of many discussions about social security. On the one hand, politicians and in particular government ministers are frequently criticised for failing to think either radically or in time-scales which extend beyond the next decade: the risks of failure and increased costs in the short term are perceived to outweigh the possibility of longer-term advantage and reform. On the other hand, teachers and researchers in the field of social security appear to be locked into the exigencies of the present and the most recent past: to be 'up-to-date' is all, because if the latest policy change (or even the possibility of change) is not acknowledged and evaluated then the contribution to understanding and policy analysis is deemed to be 'out-of-date'. This pursuit of the latest news, the most recent innovation or ministerial press release, today's statistics and tomorrow's headlines is a curse and in large measure an irrelevance to good policy analysis and a sound understanding of structures, delivery mechanisms and policy impacts. The more the subject of social policy seeks to engage with today's agenda (as it unfolds), the less it will be capable of evaluating yesterday's: it is the job of journalists to report and engage with the issues on a day-to-day basis just as it is the job of the teacher and researcher to have a longer and more detached perspective. As Kierkegaard observed, life is lived forward but understood backwards!

But students of social security, no less than policy-makers and claimants, have a right to expect appreciation of the prevailing debates and proposals. It is arguable that the pace of reform within those departments and agencies responsible for social security policy in the UK has never been greater: indeed, 'the management of change' and 'active modern service' are the central themes. But capturing the locus of reform, describing the process and doing justice to the complexity of administrative innovation are far from easy. Since the major reviews of the mid-1980s (DSS, 1985a, 1985b, 1985), policy development, the management and delivery of social security have been in perpetual motion: the 'management of change' is more than a mantra for hard-pressed officials, it is a description of an evolving reality. The dynamics of change have been driven by both push and pull factors. The former embody the imperatives of demographic change evidenced by an ageing population, a declining birth rate, a growth in lone parenthood and more reconstituted families; the traditional Beveridgean assumptions about life-time, full-time, male employment are necessarily giving way to higher rates of female labour supply, more part-time employment, more self-employment and above all more unemployment; social attitudes and political ideology are questioning the role of the state and seek to construct new partnerships between public, private and not-for-profit sectors. On the other hand, there are a number of pull factors and the significance of these changes has traditionally been much under-estimated by students of social policy; for example, there have been profoundly important changes to the structure of government departments, to their policy-making capability and management functions, to the role of Information Technology and consequently to the relationship between social security claimants and public officials. The interface between external environment and the inner world of policy-making and management is critical to an understanding of social security as the new millennium arrives.

As a background to recent policy pronouncements it is appropriate to clarify the categories and form of social security provision in the United Kingdom. The founding paradigm was cast by the Beveridge Report (1942) and it continues to cast a fading shadow. His framework gave central position to contributory benefits (following recent reforms these now include Retirement Pension, Incapacity Benefit, and Widows' Benefits and part of the Jobseeker's Allowance) which are paid for by National Insurance contributions made jointly by employees and employers. Eligibility is triggered when appropriate numbers of contributions have been made in appropriate contribution years. The number and scope of these benefits, however, have been contracting over recent years.

In contrast, the scope and significance of means- (and asset-) tested benefits have grown. For Beveridge these benefits were to be residual, providing support for those without contributions records or current entitlement to insurance benefits, the amount paid calculated according to individual/family needs and circumstances. The most significant example in the UK is Income Support (formerly called Supplementary Benefit and before that National Assistance) and is available to those without other forms of visible support. Other means-tested benefits include Housing Benefit, Council Tax Benefit, Disability Working Allowance and Family Credit. In addition, a very high proportion of payments made from the Social Fund (to meet urgent and exceptional needs and circumstances) are made to recipients of income-related benefits. Although means/asset-tested benefits 'target' benefits on particular groups they tend to be more expensive to administer, are associated with stigma and have problems of low take-up (see Chapter 6 in this volume).

Categorical benefits are neither means-tested nor insurance based, but are paid to recipients who have particular characteristics. For example, Child Benefit is paid to a designated parent or guardian (usually the mother) in respect of all children living in the UK if they are under 16 years of age, or under 19 years if in full-time education. Other examples of categorical benefits include Disability Living Allowance and Invalid Care Allowance.

Occupational benefits relate to occupational history and status. Some are paid at the discretion of employers and the obvious examples are occupational pensions; two statutory schemes, now administered by employers on behalf of the state are Statutory Sick Pay and Statutory Maternity Pay, payable on condition that employees meet specified qualifying conditions.

Finally, there are entirely discretionary payments which have been a source of considerable controversy because they provide either loans or grants to claimants (usually on Income Support) who have an urgent or exceptional need. There is no automatic right to these payments, the amount of money available is limited, and specified criteria and priorities for award vary from place to place and month to month during the financial year (see Huby and Dix, 1993).

The use of the terms means-tested (selective) and non-means-tested (universal) benefits implies a clear distinction between the two: such may have been the case in theory (and the past) but there are now no truly universal benefits. At the very least, for example, Child Benefit is only paid to families with dependent children and Retirement Pension to older people. Every benefit, to some extent or other, will be paid according to specified criteria: circumstances, contributions history or financial need. The policy challenge is to support those in need, contain cost and maintain solidarity structures by mobilising widespread consent for the underlying objectives for social security (see Chapter 2 in this volume). This is not an easy quest; indeed, it may be said to be a millennial search for the holy grail. Nevertheless, this is the challenge that successive governments have set themselves.

Social security commands a high proportion of government

expenditure and historically has been a highly contested area of public policy. It has articulated values and judgements about deserving and undeserving groups (Ditch, 1987), about the role of women and preferred family form, and it has sought to shape behaviour and reinforce social values. Some of the most fundamental concepts in social policy analysis such as universality, selectivity and stigma have been explored through studies of social security. It may be thought curious, therefore, that in recent years the ideological fault lines between left and right, at least as reflected in national policy-making, have become somewhat blurred. Peter Lilley, who was Secretary of State for Social Security between 1992 and 1997, was appointed with a reputation for radical 'new right' views and a belief that social security expenditure would be reduced. His period in office was characterised by a more thoughtful and long-term review of social security trends (and needs) than many had expected. Early government reports on the costs of social security (DSS, 1993a, 1993b) elaborated a context for reform but were predicated on questionable assumptions about growth rates, unemployment levels and demographic scenarios. They were subject to vigorous criticism (Hills, 1993) but they set a tone for rational debate which was further elaborated through a series of ministerial speeches (Lilley, 1993a, 1993b, 1995).

Providing an institutional context for this debate, however, was the fundamental reorganisation of the Department of Social Security, itself only created by the dissolving of links to the Department of Health. The Next Steps agenda, based on what may be regarded as a flawed understanding of the nature of policy-making and implementation, led to the creation of a series of semi-independent agencies responsible for the 'efficient and effective' delivery of all social security functions (see Ditch, 1993; DSS Annual Reports 1995, 1997, 1998; Ling 1994; Clarke *et al.*, 1994). Three general observations may be noted: first, far from separating and subordinating delivery issues from the policy-making function, the establishment of agencies raised the profile of front-line staff and their concerns. It is somewhat ironic that the framework documents, which set objectives and operating parameters for the new bodies, formally allowed for the Agency Chief Executives to advise and therefore help shape policy. Michael Bichard, Chief Executive of the Benefits Agency between 1991 and 1994, was especially effective in seeking to break down the practical as well as supposed theoretical divide between policy-making and policy implementation. The age of the street-level bureaucrat may not have arrived but there was a growing acknowledgement that their views and professional experience were of importance. Second, the creation of no less than five social security agencies (with a further two in Northern Ireland), working alongside the Employment Services Agency, the Inland Revenue and hundreds of local authorities did lead to evident 'boundary' disputes and territorial rivalries: the development and roll-out of the Jobseeker's Allowance is a case in point. Third, ministers became distanced from operational matters and concerns. In part, this was a convenient device to insulate themselves from uncomfortable issues. For example, would any minister want to be held directly accountable for the early and continuing problems of the Child Support Agency (CSA)? At the CSA, it may be noted, it was a series of Chief Executives who resigned or moved in rapid succession, not their ministerial masters. But the developing structure of the DSS meant that it was becoming more difficult, not easier, for ministers to effectively manage the whole system. The line management links between the ministerial team, permanent secretary and agency chief executives may have been clear on paper but were less so in practice. It is inevitable therefore that the reconfiguration of the DSS, its realignment with DFEE and local authorities in the development and delivery of significant social security benefits such as Jobseeker's Allowance, Housing Benefit and Council Tax Benefit will be an important and continuing challenge for all concerned.

If one theme of reform through the 1990s has been departmental reorganisation, a second refrain has been that of encouraging self-reliance, independence and the promotion of incentives to work. This manifests itself through debates and policy proposals in the field of pension reform and a raft of measures which seek to align receipt of benefit to work availability and employment opportunity. Mapping and monitoring these proposals and initiatives have been made more difficult because ministerial lead responsibility appears to be unclear. The rhetoric of 'joined-up-government' may convey a sense of the complex and inter-locking nature of the problems and challenges which abound in this area: in addition to the Department of Social Security, the Treasury, the DFEE, DTER, Lord Chancellor's Department, Home Office (to say nothing of Scottish and Welsh Offices and Northern Ireland Office), all have direct interests in the wider social security agenda. During the first eighteen months of the incoming Labour government it appeared as if there was no single focus for social security policy-making. Ministerial responsibility for welfare reform was vested in a junior DSS minister (Frank Field) but crucial announcements concerning lone parents, a national childcare strategy and a Working Families Tax Credit were made by the Chancellor of the Exchequer and the Secretary of State for Employment. After several months of delay the Green Paper on Welfare Reform (Cm 3805, 1998) appeared under the signature of the Prime Minister. At the first ministerial re-shuffle in July 1998 (only 14 months into office) both the Secretary of State for Social Security (Harriet Harman) and the Minister of State (Frank Field) left the government. This occasioned an opportunity for a further re-think of policy direction under the new Secretary of State, Alistair Darling, resulting in a series of consultation documents (on pensions, families, disability) and culminating in the Welfare Reform Bill published in February 1999.

The incoming Labour government were keen to make an early impact in the field of social security but were aware of the need to advance cautiously. Policy pronouncements, initiatives and innovative pilot projects all found their way on to the agenda while, at the same time a (supposedly) more radical/fundamental review of policy was undertaken. From the outset it was clear that the government had identified, to its own satisfaction, three problems inherent to the social security system: first, that poverty, inequality and social exclusion had worsened over the previous two decades and that the circumstances of families with dependent children had been especially and adversely affected; second, that social security programmes had created barriers and financial disincentives to those who might otherwise want to work; third, that there was extensive fraud and abuse in the system.

For example, within a matter of weeks of taking office, in the July 1997 budget the government announced a 'New Deal for Unemployed People' to be paid for from a windfall levy on the excess profits of the privatised utilities. The rationale was to give work, education and other opportunities to those aged 18–24 years who have been unemployed for at least six months. A so-called 'gateway' ensures that each young person in these circumstances receives an interview to assess how best to assess their skills and employment prospects. A similar 'gateway' is being developed for the longer-term unemployed who are aged over 24: already a number of initiatives provide subsidies of £75 per week for six months to employers if they recruit a long-term unemployed person; a long-term unemployed person can undertake an employment-related course of up to one year's duration whilst remaining on Jobseeker's Allowance.

At the same time the government announced a 'New Deal for Lone Parents', initially available on a pilot basis in eight areas, but 'rolled out' nationally from October 1998. The idea was to provide practical advice and support for lone parents on Income Support whose youngest child is at school and who want to work. Another announcement and one that generated considerable controversy was that the higher, lone parent rate of family premium will no longer be paid to lone parents making a new claim for Income Support, Housing Benefit, Council Tax Benefit or Jobseeker's Allowance from April 1998. Existing claimants are unaffected and lone parents already receiving the higher rate will requalify for it if they make a repeat claim or return to lone parent status after a break which does not exceed twelve weeks.

Against these policy developments Frank Field was working to prepare the proposed Green Paper on Social Security Reform. In the event, its publication was delayed by some months but when it did appear, in March 1998, eight key principles were enunciated as a guide to welfare reform. Summarised as being 'work for those who can, security for those who cannot', in full, they are as follows:

- The new welfare state should help and encourage people of working age to work where they are capable of doing so.
- The public and private sectors should work in partnership to ensure that, wherever possible, people are insured against foreseeable risks and make provision for their retirement.
- The new welfare state should provide public services of high quality to the whole community, as well as cash benefits.
- Those who are disabled should get the support they need to lead a fulfilling life with dignity.
- The system should support families and children, as well as tackling the scourge of child poverty.
- There should be specific action to attack social exclusion and help those in poverty.
- The system should encourage openness and honesty and the gateways to benefit should be clear and enforceable.
- The system of delivering modern welfare should be flexible, efficient and easy for people to use.

Undoubtedly, to date, the most coherent statement of the government's thinking about the future of social security reform, the impetus was somewhat stalled by the arrival of a new ministerial team within the DSS. The Green Paper was not dismissed, but a further and extensive round of consultation was undertaken. This involved the publication of a series of further consultation papers on families (Cm 3992), work (Cm 4102), fraud (Cm 4012) and disability (Cm 4103).

In October 1998 the government published a review of progress in respect of social security reform: *A New Contract for Welfare: Principles into Practice* (DSS, 1998h). Meanwhile, the Chancellor of the Exchequer announced a number of significant developments: for example, for those on means-tested benefits, the child personal allowance was increased by £2.50 per week from November 1998. From April 1999 the rate of

Child Benefit is to be increased by the same amount, with corresponding increases to the ordinary rate of family premium in Income Support. In itself, this represents an increase far in excess of prevailing inflation. However, it is widely expected that the next move will be to tax Child Benefit for those who pay the higher rate of income tax.

From October 1999 Family Credit and Disability Working Allowance will be replaced by a system of tax credits, payable through the wage packet with effect from April 2000. As part of this initiative there will be a Child Care Tax Credit worth 70 per cent of eligible childcare costs up to £100 for families with one child and £150 for families with two or more children.

The focus of reform has become the planning of a 'single gateway' which will redesign the way in which all people of working age will enter the benefit system. In future, they will be required to attend a interview to discuss the options available to them. In addition, the government is proposing to give more help to severely disabled people by way of a Disability Income Guarantee; to modernise Incapacity Benefit to take more account of people's ability and desire to work; and to reform Severe Disablement Allowance to provide more help for those who are disabled early in the life.

In the Social Security Bill (February 1999) the government brought forward proposals to give effect to these recommendations. In addition, they propose to establish a new 'stakeholder' pension scheme to supplement the basic Retirement Pension. The objective is to provide a second tier pension for those middle earners, about 5 million of whom do not currently have access to either occupational pensions or satisfactory private pensions and who would otherwise face poverty in their old age. Employers who did not offer access to an occupational pension would be required to support a stakeholder pension scheme. It is also proposed that pensions should be split following a divorce. This would provide additional support and financial security for women in retirement while at the same time allowing couples to make a 'clean break' at the time of divorce.

Conclusion

The present government appears to be working within a paradigm which is not greatly different to that elaborated by its predecessors. All thoughts of a 'big bang' overhaul of social security have been set aside in favour of more cautious adjustments to policy objectives and delivery systems. An over-riding sensitivity to the public perception of aggregate cost, a realisation that employment growth is limited by technological change and international competition and a capacity for rhetorical presentation over substantive innovation all suggest that past problems will return as future challenges. It is hoped that the chapters in this book will help explain why the reform of social security is neither inevitable nor easy.

References

Beveridge, W. (1942) *Social Insurance and Allied Services*, CM 6404, London: HMSO.

Clarke, J., Cochrane, J. and McLaughlin, E. (eds) (1994) *Managing Social Policy*, London: Sage.

Ditch, J. S. (1987) 'The undeserving poor: unemployed people, then and now', in M. Loney (ed.) *The State or Market Politics and Welfare in Contemporary Britain*, London: Sage, pp. 24–40.

—— (1993) 'Next Steps: restructuring the Department of Social Security', in N. Deakin and R. Page (eds) *The Costs of Welfare*, Aldershot: Avebury, pp. 64–83.

DSS (1985a) *Reform of Social Security*, vol. 1, London: HMSO.

—— (1985b) *Reform of Social Security: Programme for Change*, vol. 2, London: HMSO.

—— (1985c) *Reform of Social Security: Background Paper*, vol. 3, London: HMSO.

——(1993a) *The Growth of Social Security*, London: HMSO.

—— (1993b) *Containing the Cost of Social Security: The International Context*, London: HMSO.

—— (1995) *Social Security Departmental Report: The Government's Expenditure Plans 1995–96 to 1997–98*, London: HMSO.

—— (1997) *Social Security Departmental Report: The Government's Expenditure Plans 1997–98 to 1999–2000*, London: HMSO.

—— (1998a) *Social Security Departmental Report: The Government's Expenditure Plans 1998–99*, London: HMSO.

—— (1998b) *New Ambitions for our Country: A New Contract for Welfare*, London: HMSO.

—— (1998c) *A New Contract for Welfare: The Gateway to Work*, Cm 4102, London: HMSO.

—— (1998d) *A New Contract for Welfare: Support for Disabled People,* Cm 4103, London: HMSO.

—— (1998e) *Children First: A New Approach to Child Support*, Cm 3992, London: HMSO.

—— (1998f) *Beating Fraud is Everyone's Business: Securing the Future*, Cm 4012, London: HMSO.

—— (1998g) *New Contract for Welfare: Partnership in Pensions*, London: HMSO.

—— (1998h) *New Contract for Welfare: Principles into Practice*, London: HMSO.

Hills, J. (1993) *The Future of Welfare: A Guide to the Debate*, York: Joseph Rowntree Foundation.

10 *John Ditch*

Huby, M. and Dix, G. (1992) *Evaluating the Social Fund*, London: HMSO.

Lilley, P. (1993a) 'Benefits and costs: securing the future of social security', the Mais Lecture, mimeo.

—— (1993b) Ian Gow Memorial Lecture, 25 November.

—— (1995) Speech to the Social Market Foundation, 9 January.

Ling, T. (1994) 'The new managerialism and social security', in J. Clarke *et al.* (eds) *Managing Social Policy*, London: Sage, pp. 32–56.

1 The nature of poverty

Jonathan Bradshaw

The relief of poverty is not the only objective of social security policy. Nor is social security policy the only element of social policy to have a bearing on poverty. Nevertheless, the extent to which poverty is relieved by social security and other policies is a crucial test of their effectiveness. It is partly for this reason that poverty has always been a core preoccupation in the study of social policy. This chapter will seek to explain why poverty is important. It will then discuss the conceptual and practical difficulties involved in defining poverty. Then it will review evidence on the existence of poverty in the UK, how the level of poverty has changed in the recent past and how poverty in the UK compares with some other countries. The conclusion will briefly discuss why poverty is still a major scourge in our society and what can be done about it.

Why is poverty important?

Poverty is what philosophers describe as a *categorical need*, that is, a need which must be met in order for a person to develop properly as human being. Of course there is a good deal of debate about what constitutes a categorical need. Some philosophers do not accept that they exist at all (Barry, 1965). Some would restrict them to an 'irreducible absolutist core' – health, nutrition and shelter (Sen, 1983) and others seek to include in the idea autonomy or the capacity or freedom to choose (Doyal and Gough, 1991) or the ability to participate (Townsend, 1979). However, the essence of a categorical need is that it gives the poor a moral claim for action. As fellow human beings, we have an obligation to meet the needs of the poor. If we describe someone as poor we are saying that (subject to some reservations about the cause of their poverty and their liberty to be poor if they want to) they are in need and that their need should be met. It is therefore extremely important to use the words poor and poverty with some precision.

There are two other reasons to be preoccupied with poverty. First, poverty is not merely a problem experienced by an individual or group. We all suffer from it. Poverty is associated with all the most important problems in our society. They are problems because they affect us all. We are not just morally diminished by the sight of beggars on our streets or children undernourished or elderly people living in cold conditions. Our own lives are influenced by the fact that many of our fellow human beings are unable to flourish. Of course, the association between poverty and other social problems is not inevitable and the direction of the association is not always clear – poverty is both a cause and an effect of other problems. Indeed, poverty is commonly associated with not one but many other problems – deprivation is multiple. But an assault on poverty is an assault on many other social concerns. Indeed, it may be the most effective means of dealing with other problems. For example, it is now being argued that the main gains still to be made in the health of the nation are not going to be achieved by improving health services, or even behaving more healthily, but rather by improving the living standards of the poor and reducing stresses associated with inequalities (Quick and Wilkinson, 1991; Townsend *et al.*, 1992). To use the language of Beveridge's giants (1942); by relieving Want we can have an impact on Disease, Squalor, Ignorance and Idleness.

Second, poverty is probably the best symptom we have of the failure of our welfare state. Although not all social security policies in this country, and certainly not in other European welfare states, are concerned exclusively with poverty relief, whatever the origins and intentions of social policies, it is still the most important goal of any welfare state to reduce poverty. If a welfare state fails to do so, then it is important to find out why. Thus poverty is an outcome measure of welfare state effort and the study of poverty is an important component in helping us to understand the performance of social security systems, wider distributional arrangements and (ultimately) welfare states.

The definition of poverty

Unlike some other countries (see for example Citro and Michael, 1995) the UK has no generally accepted definition of poverty or poverty standard and (ironically) this is one reason why debate about poverty in the UK is so preoccupied with definitions. It is important to distinguish two rather different, albeit connected, debates. The first is about the concept of poverty – what it means, what it is. The second is concerned with how that concept is operationalised – how poverty is measured. The latter will be dealt with in the next section.

The main argument about the concept of poverty has centred on whether it is an *absolute* or a *relative* notion. Charles Booth (1889–1902) provided an estimate of the minimum income needed to maintain a family and used it to define those living in poverty. Seebohm Rowntree adapted Booth's methods and (perhaps wrongly, see Veit-Wilson, 1986) can be described as the father of the absolutist notion of poverty. In his first study of poverty in York (1901), Rowntree developed a poverty standard based on an estimate of the expenditure required for the maintenance of mere physical efficiency. Drawing on the newly emerging nutritional science, Rowntree formulated a diet which was required to maintain physical effort. He then priced the components of this diet, allowing for variations in consumption by women and children, at the lowest prevailing prices in York. To this he added minimal expenditure for housing, clothing and fuel. In his first study, Rowntree certainly equated poverty with physical necessities and the utmost economy was to be practised in purchasing the necessities.

Nevertheless Rowntree did not approve or advocate his poverty standard. His whole study was designed to draw attention to the plight of the poor (Veit Wilson, 1986). He followed his first study with two further studies of poverty in York in 1936 and 1950 (Rowntree, 1941; Rowntree and Lavers, 1951). It is significant that in the later studies he varied slightly from his original definition, adding a few items to the list of necessary household items which had nothing to do with physical efficiency – such as beer and tobacco. So even Rowntree, who has been acknowledged as the founder of the absolute (minimum subsistence) measure of poverty, in fact found it impossible to sustain either an absolute or purely physical standard over time.

The subsistence notion of poverty was, however, influential in policy. The calculations made by Beveridge in his report (Beveridge, 1942) were similar to Rowntree's (who was an advisor to Beveridge). These calculations with some modifications (Field, 1985; Bradshaw, 1988; Veit Wilson, 1992) formed the basis of the National Assistance Board rates set in 1948. In 1966 these became the Supplementary Benefits rates and then in 1988 they became the present Income Support rates. Over that period up to 1980 they doubled in value in real terms (in terms of prices), though they maintained a remarkably close link with average earnings (Bradshaw and Lynes, 1995). However, since 1980 they have only been linked to movements in prices and as we shall see this has been an important engine for increasing relative poverty.

In the post Second World War era few people have advocated the absolute nature of poverty. In the 1980s there was a debate between Sen (1985) and Townsend (1985) about whether absolute needs exist and from time to time conservative politicians have claimed that poverty no longer existed because basic needs had been met (ie John Moore at St Stephens Club, 11 May 1989).

When debate about poverty reemerged in the late 1950s it did so with a new conceptualisation. Subsistence notions of poverty were castigated for having false scientific pretensions, being too harsh, focused merely on physical necessities and being incapable of an understanding of poverty which encompassed both Third World and advanced societies (Townsend, 1970, 1979). The intellectual framework that moved the debate about poverty definitions forward and resolved the dilemmas inherent in understanding poverty in affluent and developing countries and over time, was the concept of relative deprivation. The relative deprivation approach to poverty, in fact, encompasses many approaches and, as we shall see, has been studied through a variety of different criteria. The essential thrust is to seek to understand what constitutes poverty in a given society. Townsend in a lifetime's work has been the father of the science of relative poverty (Townsend, 1970, 1979, 1987, 1993; Townsend *et al.*, 1987).

> Individuals, families and groups in the population can be said to be in poverty when they lack the resources to obtain the types of diet, participate in the activities and have the living conditions which are customary, or at least widely encouraged or approved, in societies to which they belong. Their resources are so seriously below those commanded by the average family or individual that they are in effect excluded from ordinary living patterns, customs and activities.
> (Townsend, 1979)

Poverty is now not merely an inability to purchase the necessities for a meagre existence but also the inability to grasp the abundance, comforts and opportunities of society. Poverty is now a dynamic concept and will vary over time and between societies. Indeed, poverty on this understanding is socially constructed, through occupational, educational, economic and other systems that establish living standards.

Before turning to the empirical challenge in trying to construct a measure which would adequately represent relative poverty, it is appropriate to introduce another rather distinct notion of poverty. This is the *Culture of poverty*, an anthropological view of poverty, ascribed to the life of the poor, and described most vividly by Oscar Lewis (1968). Poverty is seen as a culture with its own norms and values, which are distinct from those in the wider society. These norms and values in the poverty culture are pathological and, it is argued, until they are broken into by social work, psychiatry or education – no matter whatever opportunities are provided, there will be no reduction in poverty. Those who disagree with the culture of poverty thesis (Valentine, 1968) argue that, while the poor may have distinctive behaviour patterns, they are not always pathogenic. They are not the cause of poverty but the result of poverty – the determinants of poverty are to be found in the social structure, not the poor themselves.

The culture of poverty has been discussed mostly in the US context and it was an important influence on the American War on Poverty (James, 1970). In Britain echoes of the idea are sometimes found in the designation of so called 'problem estates' or poor neighbourhoods. Sir Keith Joseph might have been influenced by the notion when, as a cabinet minister, he asked the Social Research Council to undertake a programme of research on *cycles of deprivation* or *transmitted deprivation* (Rutter and Madge, 1976). More recently there has emerged a debate about the whether an *underclass* has been developing in the UK and elsewhere. In this notion there is the idea that the underclass are detached from the values, beliefs, aspirations and legal structures of society (Murray, 1984; Smith, 1992). There are also affinities with the notions of exclusion and inclusion commonly used in the European Union (Room, 1995). Nevertheless, behavioural notions of poverty do not seem to have had much impact on policies in the UK. Since Beveridge, understanding of poverty has been largely dominated by a view that the primary determinants of poverty are structural.

The measurement of poverty

Absolute definitions of poverty were operationalised using budget standards. Budget standards involve drawing up a list of commodities, employing normative judgements, supported by a combination of scientific and behavioural evidence. The budget is then priced and used as an income standard – anyone living at or below that standard is in poverty. This was the method employed by Rowntree and Beveridge and it is still used in many countries, for example, the US poverty standard was originally based on a budget standard (Orshansky, 1965) and the Swedish social assistance scales are partly determined by a normative family budget. However, in Britain they were not used in poverty research for fifty years after the Second World War. This was no doubt in part due to their association with minimum subsistence notions of poverty and in part also due to the methodological problems involved in drawing up budget standards and keeping them up to date. However, there is no reason why budget standards should not be used to represent a relative measure of poverty and the Family Budget Unit have been publishing 'modest but adequate' and 'low cost' budgets during the 1990s (Bradshaw, 1993b). Such budgets have been used to evaluate the adequacy of the Income Support and the costs of a child (Oldfield and Yu, 1993).

The first empirical study of poverty in the post-war period was *The Poor and the Poorest* (Abel-Smith and Townsend, 1965). This study was based on an analysis of the Family Expenditure Survey and employed an income standard to define poverty. The standard used was the (then) National Assistance scales plus 40 per cent. The reason for the 40 per cent margin was that families dependent on social assistance tended to have incomes above the basic scales because of disregarded earnings, income for disregarded capital and payments of 'additional requirements' for heating, special diets and other needs. *The Poor and the Poorest* was an enormously important study. It found that 14 per cent of the population were living below the standard. The government was so alarmed at this 'rediscovery of poverty' that they launched new surveys themselves – of both retirement pensioners and families which also used the same poverty standard. This 'benefit linked' poverty standard became the official definition in a series of Low Income Statistics (LIS) based on the Family Expenditure Survey and produced by the government until 1985. The series was eventually abandoned by the Conservative government in 1985, on the grounds that it was difficult to justify the standard of 40 per cent above the social assistance scales, not least because any improvement in social assistance had the effect of increasing the numbers of people defined as living in poverty. The LIS series has now been replaced by a new *Households below Average Income* (HBAI) series, which uses the same source but relates income to the average. This new poverty measure counting the number of people living below a proportion of the average (usually 50 per cent) has come to be widely employed as the poverty standard (though it is arguable that it is actually a measure of inequality).

Meanwhile academic research (but not yet official government statistics) have been preoccupied with operationalising relative poverty. Townsend (1979) was the first to seek to operationalise this approach. For a national survey of poverty carried out in 1968–69 he built up a list of sixty indicators of styles of living. He then reduced these to twelve items to form a deprivation index and for each respondent he counted the numbers lacking items on the index. He then related the distribution of those lacking items with the distribution of income and identified a threshold on the income distribution where, as income fell, the number of items lacking increased sharply. This threshold coincided with a level about 150 per cent of the then Supplementary Benefit levels. Townsend's work was subject to three particular criticisms (Piachaud, 1981, 1987). First, it was argued that there was no justification for the selection of items that made up the deprivation index; in particular, the choice was undemocratic. Second, some of those lacking items were lacking them out of choice and not because they were deprived, for example, not everyone wanted a cooked breakfast or a roast joint on Sunday (both in the selection of twelve items). Third, there was a dispute among statisticians about whether the poverty threshold that Townsend had identified actually existed (Desai, 1986; Piachaud, 1987).

In the light of these criticisms Mack and Lansley developed the social indicator methodology in the Breadline Britain Surveys in 1983 (Mack and Lansley, 1985) and 1990 (Gordon and Pantazis, 1997). Mack and Lansley drew up a list of items and then asked a sample of the population whether they considered them to be necessities. If over 50 per cent of the population considered an item to be a necessity, then it was included as a socially perceived necessity (a 'consensual' indicator of poverty). The sample were then asked whether they possessed the item and, if they did not, whether they lacked it because they could not afford it. Only those items which were lacking because they could not be afforded were included in the count of items lacking. It was notable that there was a consensus about many of the items and it was a fairly generous one, including holidays, a fridge, presents and celebrations. Furthermore in the second survey using this method (Gordon and Pantazis, 1997) the proportion of the population considering items a necessity generally increased and new items crossed the 50 per cent threshold – showing that poverty standards do change over time with rising affluence. Mack and Lansley confirmed that there was a point on the income distribution where the number of items lacking increased sharply, that coincided with an income of about 150 per cent of the Income Support level.

There is no doubt that the social indicator methods developed by Townsend and others have introduced a means of measuring poverty more directly than the methods based on indirect measures such as income. But they have not as yet been very influential on policy – indeed, it could be claimed, particularly in the last decade or so, that no research on poverty has been terribly influential. One of the problems is that politicians are able to hide behind a host of technical and other problems associated with the measurement of poverty. It is worth briefly rehearsing the nature of these.

Resources

Townsend's definition of relative poverty (above) uses the word resources. Resources imply a wider concept than income. Indeed, he pointed to the importance of *assets*, including not only goods but skills and qualifications; *fringe benefits* or *occupational welfare* such as free or subsidised meals, subsidised health care, company cars or occupational pension schemes; *income in kind* such as gifts, produce from gardens; the value of free or subsidised *public services* consumed – education, health and welfare; and the *environment*, including housing quality and the quality of the home or working environment. We have yet to establish measures that take account of all these different kinds of resources which make up a standard of living (see Bradshaw and Holmes, 1989).

Unit of analysis

There is a dilemma about what is taken as the unit of analysis in poverty studies – should it be the household, the family or the individual? Benefits are assessed on the basis of a family unit, in which it is assumed that resources are shared between a couple who support their dependants. But what about non-dependants such as adult children still living with their parents at home? Are they to be treated as independently poor even though they may be in a household which is not poor? More seriously, there is evidence (Pahl, 1989) that resources are not in fact shared equally within families and in particular between husbands and wives.

Spatial issues

Then there is a *spatial issue*, whether a poverty standard has the same value to people living in different parts of the country. The prices of commodities are not uniform in different regions – housing costs are the most obvious example, but measures of poverty tend to exclude housing costs as we shall see. Other commodities also vary in price – fuel, transport, even food. During the rapid rise in fuel prices following the oil crises in the 1970s the people on the island of Colonsay sought an increase in their social assistance scale rates to meet the extra costs of locally generated electricity. *Prices* are relevant to the measurement of poverty in another way, particularly for a poverty standard based on benefits. If benefits are increased in line with the Retail Price Index (RPI), there is no guarantee that movements in the price of commodities on which the poor spend most of their incomes – notably fuel, food and clothing will be fully reflected in the general RPI. In practice, the evidence suggests that over time the relative movement of prices have been more or less evened out (Goodman and Webb, 1995).

Equivalence

Then there is the problem of *equivalence*. The needs of families of different sizes are different and a single poverty line that does not reflect this variation in need is useless. To attempt to deal with this problem poverty standards attempt to take account of variations in need by 'equivalising' income (or expenditure) – by adjusting the standard for the numbers and ages of people in a family. There is, however, very little consensus in the literature about what is the correct equivalence scale to use – how the needs of children differ from those of adults and how economies of scale should be dealt with and a variety of different equivalent scales are in use (Buhmann *et al.*, 1988; Whiteford, 1985).

Time dimension

Then there is the *time dimension* to be considered – it is arguable that short episodes of living on a poverty income are not as serious as long-term or permanent experiences of poverty. In the former case, there is less chance that assets will run down and opportunities exist to use capital to support a previous standard of living. There is evidence that there is a good deal of turnover in the poor population and politicians have suggested that this is a reason not to be so concerned with the overall level of poverty (Lilley, 1996).

Income or expenditure?

Then there is a debate about whether *income or expenditure* is the best indirect measure of command over resources for assessing poverty. There is evidence from the Family Expenditure Survey that the expenditure of the poor is higher on average than their income and therefore expenditure might better reflect their command over resources (Blundell and Preston, 1995; Hancock and Smeaton, 1995). There is debate about the reasons for expenditure being higher than income – if it is due to borrowing and going into debt, it might be less justified to use expenditure than if it was due to dissavings or under-reporting of income.

Poverty lines and poverty gaps

Finally there is a distinction to be made between *poverty lines* and *poverty gaps*. The poverty literature tends to focus on the numbers of people living below a poverty standard or line without taking account of how much below the line they are. However, if there are a small number of people below the poverty line, but they are very far below the line, this may be more serious (and require greater transfer expenditure) than if there were a larger number of people only slightly below the poverty line. The poverty gap is a measure of the distance people are from the poverty line. A number of scholars, particularly in the comparative literature on poverty, have attempted to take account of poverty gaps as well as poverty numbers (Forster, 1993; Mitchell, 1991; Sen, 1979) but estimates of poverty gaps are very sensitive to the reliability of data on income and difficult to calculate using survey data.

All these issues are essential components of the investigation of poverty but together they can become a technical and arcane smokescreen to the essence of the subject (see also Alcock, 1993).

Poverty in the UK

What is the prevalence of poverty in the UK, who are the poor and how has poverty changed in recent years? These are the questions that will be addressed in this section. The main source of evidence used is the latest (at the time of writing) 1997 edition of *Households Below Average Income* (DSS, 1997). As we have seen, the HBAI series replaced the LIS series from 1985 and statisticians have taken the series back to 1979 on a comparable basis. The series is now published annually and, to reduce sampling errors, estimates are based on two years of the Family Expenditure Survey (though it is intended to use the Family Resources Survey in the future). The HBAI analysis has been subject to an open and systematic evaluation of the methods used and the assumptions made in respect, in particular, of such issues as what is the best equivalence scale to use, the unit of analysis employed, whether income is related to the median or mean and other technical subjects. The result of this is that the analysis in HBAI is authoritative and reliable. Nevertheless, the answer to the question 'What is the prevalence of poverty?' is inevitably 'It depends.'

Table 1.1 summarises a variety of the answers that might be produced. First it depends on which poverty threshold is used. In Table 1.1 people are defined as poor if they have equivalent income less than 60 per cent, 50 per cent and 40 per cent of national average income. The numbers counted as poor may be particularly sensitive to the

Table 1.1   The prevalence of poverty in the United Kingdom, 1994–95

Poverty standard	Individuals in benefit units	
	Number (millions)	%
Below 40% average income including the self-employed before housing costs	4.7	8
Below 40% average income excluding the self-employed before housing costs	3.3	6
Below 40% average income including the self-employed after housing costs	7.7	13
Below 40% average income excluding the self-employed after housing costs	6.0	12
Below 50% average income including the self-employed before housing costs	10.3	18
Below 50% average income excluding the self-employed before housing costs	8.3	16
Below 50% average income including the self-employed after housing costs	13.4	23
Below 50% average income excluding the self-employed after housing costs	11.4	22
Below 60% average income including the self-employed before housing costs	16.3	28
Below 60% average income excluding the self-employed before housing coasts	13.9	27
Below 60% average income including the self-employed after housing costs	18.1	32
Below 60% average income excluding the self-employed after housing costs	15.8	30

Source: Households below Average Income (DSS, 1997).

threshold chosen where there are large proportions of the population dependent on a benefit (such as Income Support or the Retirement Pension) whose level comes just below or just above a particular threshold. Second, the figures are presented including and excluding the self-employed. The rationale for this is that the incomes of the self-employed are difficult to estimate in survey research (or, indeed, for other purposes such as income tax or benefit entitlement, see Eardley and Corden, 1996), they may be understated and as the self-employed constitute 15 per cent of the bottom decile of the income distribution, including them might invalidate poverty estimates. Excluding the self-employed reduces the proportion below the income thresholds. Third, there is a debate about whether poverty should be assessed before or after housing costs have been taken into account. Housing costs are a substantial outgoing which it is not easy to vary at least in the short term. This is an argument for using the after housing costs figures. On the other hand, for mortgagees, the capital element of their payments is normally a form of investment – a resource that they might benefit from at some future time. On these grounds, income ought to be assessed before housing costs. Depending on the definition chosen, poverty would vary between 3.3 million or 6 per cent of the population and 18 million or 32 per cent of the population.

Table 1.2 explores the characteristics of the poor in terms of their economic status and their family type. It shows the proportion of each category who are poor and the risk of poverty for each group. As far as economic status is concerned, the unemployed have the highest risk of poverty with 74 per cent, then (apart from the other category) come pensioners, the self-employed and people in part-time work. The lowest risk of poverty is among households with one or two people all working full-time. The unemployed represent over a fifth of the poor (this time defined as being in the lowest quintile of equivalent income), with pensioners forming 19 per cent and the self-employed 10 per cent. In terms of family type, the highest risk of poverty is among single people with children (lone parents) where 60 per cent are poor. However, the largest single group in poverty are couples with children and in fact families with children form over half of all households in poverty.

In tracing trends in poverty since 1979 (all the series allows), again a decision has to be made about the threshold. The HBAI figures are produced in two ways. One shows trends in the proportion of the population living below a threshold held constant in real 1979 terms. Using this measure it can be seen in Table 1.3 that there were 200,000 more people in 1994–95 worse off in real terms than they had been in 1979. The problem with this standard is that, in the long term, it effectively becomes an absolute measure of poverty – fixed arbitrarily in 1979. Over the period between 1979 and 1994–95 average living standards rose by 42 per cent and the 1979 real terms measure assumes that the poor should have no share in these rising living standards. The alternative measure presented relates income to a proportion of the *contemporary* average. If the relative definition of poverty means anything, that is the most appropriate measure. In 1979 the proportion of the population in poverty by this definition was 9 per cent and by 1994–95 it had increased to 23 per cent. The family groups showing the sharpest increase were single people, lone parents and families with children. In fact, the proportion of children living in poverty increased from 10 per

Table 1.2 Characteristics of the poor

	Percentage of the bottom 20% of the income distribution in each economic status / family type including self-employed and after housing costs	Percentage of each group who have incomes below half the average including the self-employed and after housing costs (risk of poverty)
Economic status		
Self-employed	10	22
Single or couple, all in full-time work	2	2
One in full-time work, one in part-time work	1	3
One in full-time work, one not working	9	17
One or more in part-time work	10	33
Head or spouse aged over 60	19	29
Head or spouse unemployed	21	74
Other	28	61
All	100	23
Family type		
Pensioner couple	9	24
Pensioner single	8	32
Couple with children	36	22
Couple without children	9	10
Single with children	21	60
Single without children	16	22
All	100	23

Source: Households below Average Income (DSS, 1997).

cent to over 32 per cent. At the same time the increase in poverty among pensioner couples was comparatively small. All the economic status groups had an increased risk of poverty, in particular, one-earner families and part-time workers.

What are the forces that have led to this sharp increase in poverty and the unprecedented level of inequality in British society in the post-war period? They were explored by the Joseph Rowntree Foundation Inquiry (Hills, 1995, 1998). There are three broad explanations – unemployment and the increased dispersion of earnings; demographic factors;

Table 1.3 Poverty trends 1979–1994/95

	1979	1994–95 (1979 real average income)	1994–95 (contemporary average income)	% increase 1979–1994/95 (contemporary average income)
Pensioner couple	21	3	24	14
Pensioner single	12	4	32	167
Couple with children	8	10	22	175
Couple without children	5	5	10	100
Single with children	19	18	60	215
Single without children	7	13	23	229
Self-employed	15	15	22	47
Single or couple, all in full-time work	1	1	2	100
One in full-time work, one in part-time work	1	1	3	200
One in full-time work, one not working	4	4	17	325
One or more in part time work	15	14	33	120
Head or spouse aged 60 or over	20	4	29	45
Head or spouse unemployed	58	46	74	28
Other	35	24	61	74
All (%)	9	9	23	156
All (millions)	5	5.2	13.4	168

Source: Households below Average Income (DSS, 1997).

Note: Individuals below 50 per cent average income including the self-employed after housing costs.

and changes in social and fiscal policies which have left the state much less capable of mitigating poverty and reducing inequalities.

The most obvious economic factor is that labour demand has not kept pace with labour supply. Male full-time jobs have fallen by over two million since 1979. Female full-time jobs have increased slightly. Overall, there has been a shift from full-time to part-time jobs: part-time jobs have increased by over two million since 1979. Jobs have become less secure, more episodic and casual. There has been a sharp increase in self-employment and self-employed people have a much wider dispersion of income than those in employment. Although overall more people are in employment as a result of the increase in part-time work, that work is concentrated in fewer households. One in seven households had no working person in 1993 compared with one in 20 in the mid-1970s. In contrast, the proportion of households with two earners increased from 52 per cent to 61 per cent between 1975 and 1993.

The other economic factor is that earnings have become more dispersed. In 1990 the relativities between men's earnings were higher than at any time during this century. There has been a rapid increase in low pay and a stretching of the earnings between skilled and unskilled workers, less well educated and more educated people, young people and others and, of course, huge increases at the top of the scale. Female earnings have come to play a more important part in living standards and in keeping families out of poverty. Without women's earnings Harkness *et al.* (1994) have estimated that poverty rates among couples with children would be 50 per cent higher.

The demographic factors include the increase in the number of elderly people in the population. Although on average the living standards of pensioners have improved over the period, thanks largely to the increase in the proportion benefiting from occupational pensions or the state earnings related pension scheme, the incomes of pensioners have become more dispersed with older, single, female pensioners in particular becoming relatively worse off. The growth in unemployment has in part been the result of demographic factors – particularly the large birth cohorts of the 1960s seeking employment in a tight labour market. Finally poverty has been exacerbated by the growth in the numbers of lone parent families as a result of the breakdown of marriage and cohabitation and the increase in births outside marriage (Ford and Millar, 1998). Fewer lone mothers have been able to get access to the labour market and the proportion dependent on Income Support has risen (Bradshaw *et al.*, 1996).

Included among the policy measures that have contributed to the increase in poverty was the decision in 1980 to break the link between the uprating of some benefits and earnings (Bradshaw and Lynes, 1995); the abolition of some benefits in particular for 16–18-year-olds, students, the long-term unemployed and lone parents; the emasculation of the school meals service; the substantial shift from direct to indirect taxation and large increases in VAT; and real cuts in expenditure on some services, most dramatically the housing programme and housing subsidies with a resulting rapid increase in real rents.

How does poverty in Britain compare?

Successive government spokesmen have sought to argue that this increased poverty and inequality is not unique to Britain – the natural consequences of international competition or the necessary concomitant of deregulation required to enable the UK 'to lead the world out of recession'. The JRF Inquiry showed that the increase in inequality in the UK was second only to New Zealand during the 1980s (Barclay, 1995; Hills, 1995). Table 1.4, based on the data from the Luxembourg

Table 1.4   Percentage of households with equivalent income below 50 per cent average after social security benefits and direct taxation, *c.* 1990

	Aged (S).	Aged (C)	Single (NC)	Couple (NC)	Lone Parent	Couple (CH)	Other	Total
AUS	50.2	22.2	24.8	7.2	57.1	10.9	13.2	19.7
BEL	12.4	11.4	9.2	5.1	9.4	4.7	6.2	7.1
CAN	8.9	4.4	27.1	7.5	48.6	10.8	15.2	15.1
CZE	4.0	0.8	4.5	0.7	9.9	1.1	3.0	2.1
DEN	8.8	2.8	17.7	2.7	6.5	3.1	4.7	8.2
FIN	23.1	3.0	18.5	3.6	6.3	2.8	5.4	9.6
GER	21.7	12.9	21.7	16.3	34.2	12.1	16.9	17.5
HUN	22.2	10.5	21.3	6.9	6.9	7.2	17.4	11.4
ISR	35.6	22.1	20.1	9.0	34.4	19.5	18.7	20.0
ITA	9.0	4.1	7.4	7.8	4.9	14.6	11.6	9.6
NET	3.8	7.6	18.1	5.6	27.4	8.0	5.4	9.3
NOR	16.5	1.5	15.3	0.6	12.9	2.1	1.3	8.2
POL	18.6	12.4	10.1	7.6	6.7	15.4	14.7	13.1
RUS	83.1	37.9	52.0	25.2	37.4	19.5	33.3	34.3
SPA	16.3	20.8	23.5	12.2	27.7	15.0	17.1	16.0
SLO	1.8	0.5	5.7	1.5	7.9	1.7	2.2	2.2
SWE	9.6	0.7	18.3	2.0	2.6	2.9	0.0	9.1
TWN	49.0	42.5	19.2	13.4	25.0	14.6	19.1	17.5
UK	46.5	30.4	23.5	8.9	51.8	17.5	17.8	23.0
USA	40.5	17.0	26.2	9.2	53.9	18.4	33.8	23.5
AVG	24.1	13.3	19.2	7.6	23.6	10.1	12.9	13.8

Source: Bradshaw and Chen (1997).

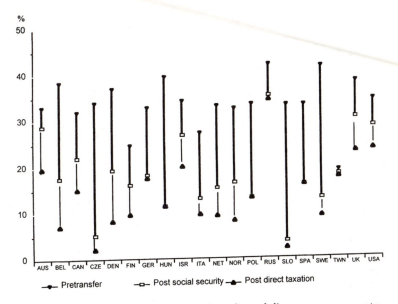

Figure 1.1 The impact of social security benefits and direct taxes on poverty rates

Income Survey (Bradshaw and Chen, 1997), shows that after transfers, out of twenty countries, the UK (in 1991) had the third highest overall poverty rate after the USA and Russia. The figure of 23.0 per cent of poor households is nearly double the average for all countries. The UK also has an above average poverty rate for all household groups. It has the third highest rate of poverty among lone parent families and aged couples and the fourth highest rate for couples with children and aged singles.

Figure 1.1 compares the performance of different countries in reducing poverty. Of the twenty countries the Czech Republic and Slovakia are most successful (but not necessarily most efficient), reducing over 90 per cent of their pre-transfer poverty. Taiwan is the least successful, reducing just over 7 per cent of their pre-transfer poverty. The UK is fourth least successful after Taiwan, Russia and the USA, reducing just 40 per cent of its pre-transfer poverty. Figure 1.1 also shows that in the UK the respective contribution to poverty reduction made by social security benefits and direct taxes is fairly even. In most other countries most of the reduction in poverty occurs as a result of social security benefits.

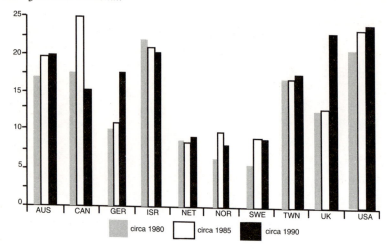

Figure 1.2   Households below 50 per cent average income after transfers

At the time of writing there are ten countries in the LIS data set with data for all three sweeps – *circa* 1979, 1985 and 1990. For these countries it is possible to compare trends in poverty and inequality over time. Figure 1.2 summarises trends in poverty for these ten countries over the decade. There has been an increase in poverty rates in all countries except Israel and Canada over this period but by far the sharpest increase in poverty has occurred in the UK where between 1979 and 1991. Only Germany experienced anything near this level of increase.

If account had been taken of housing costs, services in kind and indirect taxes there is some evidence from previous comparative analyses that the position of the UK might not be considered as bad (Saunders, 1992; Smeeding *et al.*, 1993; Whiteford and Kennedy, 1995). Also Ramprakash (1994) and Zaidi and de Vos (1996) found that if household expenditure was used instead of income then the UK had comparatively lower poverty rates. If other elements of poverty had been included – poverty gaps, or some kind of aggregate measure of poverty, as developed by Sen (1979), again there is previous evidence that the UK would not appear to do so badly (Forster, 1993; Mitchell, 1991).

Nevertheless, the comparative position of the UK appears to have deteriorated from that in the *circa* 1980 and *circa* 1985 LIS sweeps. This confirms previous work (Atkinson *et al.*, 1995; Bradshaw, 1991; Mitchell, 1991). Also the relative position of the UK is rather worse in 1991 than the European Commission found in the late 1980s (Hagenaars *et al.*, 1994; Ramprakash. 1994). The fact that in the UK poverty is relatively worse after the impact of direct taxes and social security benefits indicates that its position is not just determined by market forces, international competition or other external factors which affect the primary distribution but also by the comparative failure of our social and fiscal policies to protect the poor against the impact of those forces.

Conclusion

A number of attempts have been made to review the evidence of the impact of increasing poverty particularly for families with children (Bradshaw, 1990; Kumar, 1993; Wilkinson, 1994). Since the early 1980s some indicators of outcome show improvements despite the increase in poverty – thus general educational attainment has improved (but there is evidence that reading standards among 7- and 8- year-olds deteriorated during the 1980s). Despite common prejudice, teenage crime has fallen, as has smoking among children and adolescents. Some indicators show improvement, though at a slower rate than might be expected in comparison with other countries, for example, infant mortality, child mortality and morbidity. Certainly there is no evidence that differentials in infant mortality have narrowed, indeed strong evidence that the association between deprivation and poor health has strengthened (Phillimore *et al.*, 1994).

There is no doubt that some things have got worse. Homelessness has increased sharply and many families with dependent children and young people have had to spend time in temporary, mostly bed and breakfast accommodation with adverse effects on their health and their children's education and development. Housing conditions have deteriorated particularly for those poor families living in inner city areas in run-down estates and in high rise flats, often in damp dwellings which are difficult and expensive to heat adequately. There is also evidence that childhood morbidity has increased and it is also probable that children's diets have deteriorated which may explain the levelling off in the improvement of children's heights in the late 1980s. Drug offenders between the ages of 17 and 29 doubled in number during the 1980s and deaths from solvent abuse increased fourfold. The suicide rate among young men increased by 75 per cent between 1983 and 1990. The number of children on the child protection registers increased fourfold in the 1980s and the number of children in care has increased since the mid-1980s. There is no doubt that the quality of life in economically deprived neighbourhoods in the inner cities has got worse over time and poverty has become more spatially concentrated in these areas and these areas suffer more from poor health, crime, drug abuse, depression and other social problems.

What can be done to reduce these very high levels of poverty in the UK? Here is not the place to rehearse a full anti-poverty agenda but the number one priority must be to improve the living standards of poor families with children. To this end we await the introduction of the statutory minimum wage, good quality and affordable childcare, more generous in-work benefits for children, including a further increase in child benefits, a substantial increase in Income Support and Housing Benefit for families with children. These policies call for, indeed inevitably involve, increasing the level of taxation on those who are better off and have access to the labour market.

Note

Material from the Family Expenditure Survey is Crown Copyright; has been made available by the Office for National Statistics through the ESRC Data Archive; and has been used by permission. Neither the Office of National Statistics nor the ESRC Data Archive bear any responsibility for the analysis or the interpretation of the data reported here.

References

Abel Smith, B. and Townsend, P. (1965) *The Poor and the Poorest*, Occasional Papers in Social Administration, London: Bedford Square Press.

Alcock, P. (1993) *Understanding Poverty*, London: Macmillan.

Atkinson A. B. *et al.* (1995) *Income Distribution in OECD Countries: Evidence from the Luxembourg Income Study*, Paris: OECD.

Atkinson, A. B. and Micklewright, J. (1992) *Economic Transformation in Eastern Europe and the Distribution of income*. Cambridge: Cambridge University Press.

Barclay, P. (1995) *Income and Wealth*, vol. 1, York: Joseph Rowntree Foundation.

Barry B. (1965) *Political Argument*, London: Routledge and Kegan Paul.

Beveridge Report (1942) *Social Insurance and Allied Services*, Cmd 6404, London: HMSO.

Blundell, R. and Preston, I. (1995) *Income, Expenditure and the Living Standards of the UK Households*,

Booth, C. (1889–1902) *Life and Labour of the People of London*, London: Macmillan.

Bradshaw, J. (1988) 'Welfare benefits', in R. Walker and G. M. Parker (eds) *Money Matters: Income, Wealth and Financial Welfare*, London: Sage Publications.

—— (1990) *Child Poverty and Deprivation in the UK*, London: National Children's Bureau.

—— (1991) 'Audit of an era: the impact on inequality of social policies under Thatcher', in P. Saunders and S. Graham (eds) *Beyond Economic Rationalism: Alternative Futures for Social Policy*, Social Policy Research Centre: Reports and Proceedings, Sydney: University of New South Wales.

—— (1993a) 'Developments in social security policy', in C. Jones (ed.) *New Perspectives on the Welfare State in Europe*, London: Routledge.

—— (ed) (1993b) *Budget Standards for the UK*, Aldershot: Avebury.

Bradshaw, J. *et al.* (1996) *The Employment of Lone Parents: A Comparison of Policy in 20 Countries*, London: Family Policy Studies Centre.

Bradshaw, J. and Chen, J.-R. (1997) 'Poverty in the UK: a comparison with nineteen other countries', *Benefits* 1–97.

Bradshaw, J. and Holmes, H. (1989) *Living on the Edge*, London: Child Poverty Action Group.

Bradshaw, J. and Lynes, T. (1995) *Benefit Uprating Policy and Living Standards*, Social Policy Reports Number 1, Social Policy Research Unit, York: University of York.

Bradshaw, J. and Millar, J. (1991) *Lone Parent Families in the UK*, London: HMSO.

Buhmann, B. *et al.* (1988) 'Equivalence scales, well-being, inequality and poverty: sensitivity estimates across ten countries using the Luxembourg Income Survey database', *The Review of Incomes and Wealth*, June, 115–141.

Citro, C. F. and Michael, R. T. (1995) (eds) *Measuring Poverty: A New Approach*, Washington, DC: National Academy Press.

Department of Social Security (1997) *Households Below Average Income: A Statistical Analysis 1979–1994/95*, London: HMSO.

Desai, M. (1986) 'Drawing the line: on defining the poverty threshold', in P. Golding (ed.) *Excluding the Poor*, London: Child Poverty Action Group.

Doyal, L. and Gough, I. (1991) *A Theory of Human Need*, London: Macmillan.

Eardley, T, and Corden, A. (1996) *Low Income Self Employment*, Studies in Cash and Care, Aldershot: Avebury/Gower.

Field, F. (1985) *What Price a Child?*, London: Policy Studies Institute.

Ford, R. and Millar, J. (eds) (1998) *Private Lives and Public Responses: Lone Parenthood and Future Policy in the UK*, London: PSI.

Forster, M. (1993) *Comparing Poverty in 13 OECD Countries: Traditional and Synthetic Approaches*, Income Study Working Paper No. 100, Luxembourg: CEPS/INSTEAD.

Goodman, A. and Webb, S. (1995) *The Distribution of UK Household Expenditure 1979–92*, Commentary No. 49, London: Institute of Fiscal Studies.

Gordon, D. and Pantazis, C. (1997) *Breadline Britain in the 1990s*, Aldershot: Avebury/Gower.

Hagenaars, A. *et al.* (1994) *Poverty Statistics in the Late 1980s: Research Based on Micro Data*, Luxembourg: Eurostat.

Hancock, R. and Smeaton, D. (1995) *Pensioners' Expenditure: An Assessment of Changes in Living Standards 1979–1991*, London: Age Concern Institute of Gerontology, Kings College.

Harkness, S. *et al.* (1994) *Women, Low Pay and Family Income Inequality*, STICERD, London: London School of Economics.

Hills, J. (1995) *Joseph Rowntree Foundation Inquiry into Income and Wealth*, vol. 2: *A Summary of Evidence*, York: Joseph Rowntree Foundation.

—— (1998) *Income and Wealth: The Latest Evidence*, York: Joseph Rowntree Foundation.

James, E. (1970) *America Against Poverty*, London: Routledge and Kegan Paul.

Kumar, V. (1993) *Poverty and Inequality in the UK: The Effects on Children*, London: National Children's Bureau.

Lewis, O. (1968) 'Culture of poverty', in D. Moynihan (ed.) *On Understanding Poverty: Perspectives from the Social Sciences*, New York: Basic Books.

Lilley, P. (1996) 'Equality, generosity and opportunity – welfare reform and Christian values', speech delivered at Southwark Cathedral, 13 June.

Mack, J. and Lansley, S. (1985) *Poor Britain*, London: Allen and Unwin.

Mitchell, D. (1991) *Income Transfers in Ten Welfare States*, Aldershot: Avebury.

Moore, J. (1989) *The End of the Line for Poverty*, London: Conservative Political Centre.

Murray, C. (1984) *Losing Ground*, New York: Basic Books Inc.

Oldfield, N. and Yu, A. C. S. (1993) *The Cost of a Child: Living Standards for the 1990s*, London: Child Poverty Action Group.

Orshansky, M. (1965) 'Counting the poor: another look at the poverty profile', *Social Security Bulletin* 28 (3).

Pahl, J. (1989) *Money and Marriage*, London: Macmillan.

Phillimore, P., Beattie, A. and Townsend, P. (1994) 'Widening inequality of health in northern England 1981–1991', *British Medical Journal*, 308, 1125–1128.

Piachaud, D. (1981) 'Peter Townsend and the Holy Grail', *New Society*, 10 September.

Piachaud, D. (1987) 'Problems in the definition and measurement of poverty', *Journal of Social Policy* 16(2): 125–146.

Quick, A. and Wilkinson, R. (1991) *Income and Health*, London: Socialist Medical Association.

Ramprakash, D. (1994) 'Poverty in the countries of the European Union: a synthesis of Eurostat's statistical research on poverty', *Journal of European Social Policy*, 4(2): 117–129.

Room, G. (ed.) (1995) *Beyond the Threshold: The Measurement and Analysis of Social Exclusion*, Cambridge: The Polity Press,

Rowntree, B. S. (1901) *Poverty: A Study of Town Life*, London: Longmans.

—— (1941) *Poverty and Progress*, London: Longmans, Green and Co.

Rowntree, S. and Lavers, G. R. (1951) *Poverty and the Welfare State*, London: Longmans, Green and Co.

Rutter, M. and Madge, N. (1976) *Cycles of Disadvantage: A Review of Research*, London: Heinemann.

Saunders, P. (1992) 'The social wage in international perspective', *SPRC Newsletter*.

Sen, A. K. (1979) 'Issues in the measurement of poverty', *Scandinavian Journal of Economics* 81, 285–307.

—— (1983) 'Poor, relatively speaking', *Oxford Economic Papers* 35: 135–169.

—— (1985) 'A sociological approach to the measurement of poverty: a reply to Professor Peter Townsend', *Oxford Economic Papers* 37: 669–676.

Smeeding, T. *et al.* (1993) 'Poverty, inequality and family living standards impacts across seven nations: the effects of non cash subsidies for health, education and housing', *The Review of Income and Wealth*, series 39, no 3, 229–256.

Smith, D. (ed.) (1992) *Understanding the Underclass*, London: Policy Studies Institute.

Townsend, P. (1970) *The Concept of Poverty*, London: Heinemann.

—— (1979) *Poverty in the United Kingdom*, Harmondsworth: Allen Lane and Penguin Books.

—— (1985) 'A sociological approach to the measurement of poverty: a rejoinder to Professor Amartya Sen', *Oxford Economic Papers* 37: 659–668.

—— (1987) 'Deprivation', *Journal of Social Policy* 16(2): 125–146.

—— (1993) *The International Analysis of Poverty*, Milton Keynes: Harvester Wheatsheaf.

Townsend, P., Corrigan, P. and Kowarzik, U. (1987) *Poverty and Labour in London: Interim Report of the Centenary Survey*, London: Low Pay Unit.

United Nations (1995) *The Copenhagen Declaration and Programme of Action: World Summit for Social Development 6–12 March 1995*, New York: United Nations Publications.

Valentine, C. (1968) *Culture and Poverty*, Chicago: University of Chicago Press.

Veit-Wilson, J. H. (1986) 'Paradigms of poverty: a rehabilitation of B. S. Rowntree', *Journal of Social Policy* 15(1): 69–99.

—— (1992) 'Muddle or mendacity? The Beveridge Committee and the poverty line', *Journal of Social Policy* 16(2): 183–211

Whiteford, P. (1985) *A Family's Needs: Equivalence Scales, Poverty and Social Security*, Research Paper No. 27, Canberra: Department of Social Security.

Whiteford, P. and Kennedy, S. (1995) *Incomes and Living Standards of Older People*, Department of Social Security Research Report 43, London: HMSO.

Wilkinson, R. (1994) *Unfair Shares: The Effects of Widening Income Differences on the Welfare of the Young*, London: Barnados.

Zaidi, M.A. and de Vos, K. (1996) 'Trends in consumption-based poverty and inequality in the member states of the European Community', paper presented to the 24th General Conference of the International Association of Research on Income and Wealth, Lillehamer, Norway, 18–24 August 1996, mimeo.

2 The aims of social security

Roy Sainsbury

Introduction

It is misleading to talk about the 'aims of social security' as if they are something that exist on their own, providing a set of universal criteria against which we can evaluate the social security system now or at any given time in the past. The reality is that the aims of social security are constantly changing; sometimes in slow, almost imperceptible, ways as policy develops in a familiar incremental fashion and sometimes in big steps as major reviews of the benefit system take place or as new governments take office.

There are a number of problems in addressing the question of the aims of social security. The social security system at present comprises around thirty different benefits that have grown in a somewhat piece-meal fashion over the most of this century (Hill, 1990). Many are familiar and huge in scope – retirement pensions, Income Support, Child Benefit. Others are also well known though may affect fewer people – sickness benefit, Family Credit, and the range of disability benefits. Each of these benefits has its origins in legislation passed at some stage this century. Some, like pensions and benefits for unemployed people, date from before the First World War. Others, like many of the range of disability benefits, are the product of more recent times. At some point, however, each benefit will have had an initial purpose or purposes – its aims. The problem is that these initial aims are not always easy to pin down, however hard we scrutinise public documents and speeches (notwithstanding the possibility that other, indirect or covert aims, might also exist). We are often left therefore trying to recreate the aims of individual benefits from the evidence available. If this task could be achieved we would have thirty or more different lists of aims (which also would be one interpretation only; others would be possible) rather than something we could confidently say represented the 'aims of social security' as a whole.

One way of making sense of the task is to reformulate the question, and ask what are the aims (social, economic or whatever) that are being pursued through the medium of social security policy. Social security is just one of many instruments of policy that can be used to pursue the wider aims of government. Those outside government will also seek to promote their own (often conflicting) aims by trying to influence the content of social security policy. In this chapter we will describe some of the main aims that people inside and outside government have pursued using social security as a vehicle for policy. We will see that social security is a potentially powerful and flexible tool. This flexibility derives from the fact that it delivers welfare mainly in the medium of money, rather than in goods and services, in a society based on the operation of the market economy in which money is essential for the maintenance of individual welfare. However, social security is also often cumbersome, unwieldy and unsuccessful. Its rules and regulations, contained in primary and secondary legislation, are many and complex and not amenable to rapid revision in the face of social and economic change.

This chapter is concerned with *aims*. This is a deliberate choice. We could have chosen to discuss the functions of social security, in the sense of what social security actually does and what its outcomes are.[1] However, this approach would have hidden, or at best obscured, the importance of the political nature of social security. As we shall see, social security can be used for the relief of poverty. It has explicitly been used in this way in the past, and we can therefore say that the relief of poverty *has been* an aim of social security. But we would be wrong to say that one of the aims of social security *is* always the relief of poverty. It is also true that one effect of social security policy (together with the tax and National Insurance systems) has been to transfer resources to those with little or no money. But again we cannot say that the redistribution of wealth *is* an aim of social security. Aims are chosen and that choice is essentially political in nature.

The approach taken in this chapter is to describe aims that have been pursued using social security policy. In doing so an attempt will be made to identify who has been, and is, associated with each aim. What will emerge from our review will be a picture of the aims of social security being constantly contested, defined and redefined, invented and reinvented, taken up and abandoned. We will also see how the aims that are identified are seldom one-dimensional; it is usually the case that a number of aims are being pursued at once, or that aims are qualified or restricted by constraints. Aims will also overlap and support each other, on the one hand, and contradict each other, on the other.

We will also see that there is a useful distinction to be made between some of the long-standing aims that have been associated with the social security system and more recent attempts to use the benefit system to pursue new and wider aims. We will begin our review with the former.

Old and familiar aims

The relief of poverty?

Perhaps one of the most commonly held perceptions about the social security system in this country is that, whatever else it does, social security is there primarily to relieve poverty. Such a view is not surprising given that many of the main benefits can only be claimed by people with low incomes or without any other source of income at all. Certainly the relief of poverty as an aim would have been recognisable to the architects of the benefits introduced early in this century, and also by readers of the Beveridge Report (Beveridge, 1942).

That the state has a duty to relieve poverty among its citizens has been recognised in legislation since Elizabethan times (Fraser, 1973). The first revolution in the provision for the poor and destitute took place over 200 years later with the introduction of the Poor Law Reform Act of 1834. The Poor Law was still in existence in the first decade of this century but was increasingly recognised as inappropriate for sections of the population whose poverty could not be blamed on idleness and fecklessness but on the inevitability of old age and the contingencies of unemployment and sickness. The first piece of legislation which is recognisably part of what we now describe as the social security system was the Old Age Pensions Act of 1908. Like much social legislation it was essentially an answer to a problem. The problem was that of poverty among the population of old people in the country (George, 1968; Thane, 1982). The main aim of old age pensions, which has often been cited as one of the central aims of social security as a whole, was therefore the relief of poverty. The aim of unemployment and sickness insurance is perhaps better described as poverty prevention than the relief of poverty. Poverty was often the result of losing employment or losing pay through sickness. By paying benefits to people soon after suffering a temporary reduction or loss of earnings, the intention was to stop people sliding into poverty in the first place rather than helping when they were there.

Beveridge (1942) recognised that the main causes of poverty among those below retiring age were the interruption or loss of earnings through sickness and unemployment. His plan for a system of social insurance and social assistance benefits was explicitly designed to conquer what he graphically described as the Giant of Want. Poverty was recognised as a social evil which could strike anyone and which everyone had an interest in alleviating. However, even fifty years later it is arguable whether the relief of poverty is prominent today as an aim of social security (see Chapter 3).

In the policy pronouncements of successive Conservative Secretaries of State for Social Security since 1979 the relief of poverty was not cited as an explicit aim of social security. Indeed, one would be hard pressed to find any reference to poverty at all. The word all but disappeared from the discourse of government. This is not the result of fad or fashion. Recent governments have refused to engage in a debate about the adequacy of social security benefits, particularly of income support, the main social assistance benefit (Bradshaw and Lynes, 1995). To accept that poverty exists is to accept that it can be identified and measured, and that an adequate level of income can be defined that represents when poverty is no longer present. So in order to evade a discussion about adequacy, the language of poverty has been denied. However, as we mentioned in the introduction, the effect of providing social security benefits to people with little or no other income is always to ameliorate poverty, even when one chooses to ignore its existence.

It seems reasonable to say that the relief of poverty has been an explicit and recognisable aim of social security for most of this century. For many outside government the relief of poverty remains *the* aim of social security. For those inside government between 1979 and 1997 a different aim gained ascendancy – the *meeting of need*, to which we now turn our attention.

Meeting needs

Meeting people's needs is often claimed as one of the aims of social security. As a broad statement of intent there are probably few who would disagree. However, what 'meeting people's needs' translates to in concrete policies is the stuff of politics, open to debate and fundamental disagreement. What needs are we talking about? Whose needs should be met? How, and to what extent, should those needs be met? There are no clear or right answers although, of course, the government of the day has the power to provide the answers at least for a limited time. Those outside government will try perhaps to get new needs recognised and met or argue that some needs should be met from somewhere other than the social security system.

There are numerous examples in the history of the benefits system of new needs generating a response through social security policy. The introduction of family allowances in 1945 (subsequently reformed and renamed Child Benefit in 1977) in recognition of the problems caused by low incomes in general and for large families in particular is one example (Brown, 1984; Hall *et al.*, 1975; Macnicol, 1980). In the late 1960s the needs of disabled people were systematically and comprehensively catalogued in surveys by the then Office of Population Censuses and Surveys. Prominent among the needs identified were for help with the tasks of everyday living, supervision during the day or night and assistance with getting about from place to place. The extra financial burden that these needs placed on disabled people and their families and carers was also recognised as requiring a response from government. Hence, in the early 1970s the attendance and mobility needs of disabled people were explicitly addressed in the introduction of two new benefits, Attendance Allowance and Mobility Allowance.[2]

Even when needs are recognised the way in which they are addressed can show marked variations. Within the social assistance schemes in this country since the Second World War,[3] there have been provisions for meeting claimants' needs for essential and substantial items of household furniture and equipment that they could not otherwise afford. Until 1988 these were in the form of lump-sum payments (extra needs payments under the Supplementary Benefit scheme and single payments under Income Support) or enhancements to weekly benefit rates. However, since 1988 grants have largely been replaced by *loans* from the cash-limited Social Fund which have to be repaid from benefit income. Are people's needs still being met? The answer can only be heavily qualified: yes for some, but possibly only at the cost of creating other needs elsewhere in their lives, and no for others who are refused help because their need does not have a high enough priority (according to the rules of the Social Fund) or because there is simply no money left in the budget regardless of their need (Huby and Dix, 1992).

This discussion of meeting needs developed from the earlier discussion of the relief of poverty. The two are clearly linked in that relieving poverty is one manifestation of meeting need – the need for a subsistence income to avoid destitution. But needs arise in a variety of contexts as we have seen in relation to disability and the Social Fund. To what extent, then, can we say that meeting need is an aim of social security? As with the relief of poverty it is probably fair to say that it has been an aim in the past but we do not find it stated explicitly now. The reason may be that 'meeting need' (like the relief of poverty) implies a commitment to defining and measuring need and devising social security benefits paid at sufficient amounts to meet that need. We now find that 'helping to meet need' is more likely to be found since 'helping' takes the responsibility for 'meeting' need away from the DSS and places it back with the individual. And as we shall see later, 'encouraging personal responsibility' *is* a current aim of the social security system.

Income maintenance and replacement

So far we have discussed the relief of poverty and meeting needs as two aims of social security and seen the overlap between them. However, social security has not only been used in this country as a safety net, providing social assistance to those with no other means of supporting themselves. Social security has also had the function of helping maintain the circumstances of people and their families at times when they may suffer an interruption of earnings. This is the basis of the *contributory* benefits in the social security system (such as sickness, maternity and unemployment benefits). By definition, eligibility for these benefits depends on contributions made through the National Insurance scheme, and not on a test of means. They have been traditionally called the 'short-term benefits' which indicates clearly the original intention behind them – to provide a stopgap income between periods of employment.

Although, in short-term benefits we can identify the social security system providing something different from the social assistance benefits, is it also possible to identify a separate set of aims behind them? Part of the answer can be traced to the introduction of the National Insurance scheme at the beginning of the century. At that time breadwinners with no savings or assets behind them were likely to commence a rapid descent into poverty if they lost their earnings through unemployment or sickness. As we have described earlier, the Poor Law was increasingly recognised as an unsatisfactory and inappropriate response to this group of people. The answer to this problem devised by the government of Lloyd George (and introduced in 1911) drew heavily on the German model of social insurance which was based on contributions made by workers, employers and government (Fraser, 1973). Contributions entitled unemployed and sick workers to a flat-rate benefit for a fixed period of time. However, despite the innovation of insurance funding, the aim of the benefits can still be expressed in terms of preventing poverty or meeting the needs of unemployed or sick workers. Similarly, although state retirement pensions are based on National Insurance contributions and are a form of income replacement rather than maintenance, their original aim was the prevention of poverty.

The aim of maintaining a household's circumstances is also present in those aspects of the social security system concerned with housing. Rent rebates paid to local authority tenants and rent allowances paid to private sector tenants help people maintain their accommodation when they lose the means of paying for it. Mortgage interest payments for house-owning Income Support recipients ameliorate the problem of making payments during unemployment, although provisions have become less generous in recent years and individual claimants now bear more of the burden for protecting their mortgages than in the past.

Compensation

The Workmen's Compensation Act of 1897 gave a limited number of manual workers employed in dangerous occupations rights to lump-sum compensatory payments from their employers if they suffered injury from an accident at work (Thane, 1982). Before 1897 the injured worker had to rely on the common law of negligence for any kind of remedy, which involved the costly and difficult exercise of proving that the employer was to blame for the accident. By the time of the Second World War, problems with the operation of the Act (particularly the practices of some insurance companies) led to calls for reform. When a Royal Commission, set up in 1938, was abandoned at the outbreak of war, the task of reviewing workmen's compensation fell to Beveridge, who recommended a state-run industrial injuries scheme to remove employers and insurance companies from the determination and administration of payments. The new scheme, along the lines suggested by Beveridge, was implemented in 1948, and it is by this route that *compensation* has found a place among the functions of social security. Today, the basis for determining an award of Industrial Injuries Disablement Benefit is the same as it was in 1948. Payments are made on the basis of an assessment of the degree of disablement suffered by the claimant, and not related to means (i.e. not connected to the relief of poverty) nor to the claimant's needs (Brown, 1982).

From the perspective of the 1990s the role of compensation played by this part of the social security system stands somewhat apart from other benefits which provide income maintenance and replacement and are mostly aimed at people with low levels of other income. Therefore, while we can say that social security does in practice provide compensation, there is little evidence to say that this is a recognised aim of social security. What evidence there is (for example, in the legislative changes implemented in 1988 which stopped benefits to people with low levels of disablement) suggests that compensation is not now viewed as a legitimate aim or function of the social security system.

Redistribution

One of the effects of implementing social security policies is to redistribute financial resources between groups of the population. Money collected through taxation and National Insurance contributions is allocated to people on the basis of the rules and regulations of social security legislation. It is possible to identify a number of ways in which resources are redistributed, for example: from rich to poor ('vertical redistribution' between income groups); from those in work to the unemployed, from people without children to families (an example of 'horizontal redistribution') from people of working age to retired people; from the healthy to the sick.

We can see therefore that redistribution is an effect of social security, but can we say that it is also an aim? The answer is that it could be, but it is perhaps better to view redistribution as the inevitable consequence of trying to meet other aims such as relieving poverty or meeting needs. If you want to achieve these aims you have to take money from one source to transfer it to the target population. So, redistribution cannot be avoided. Of course, it is possible to treat redistribution as an end in itself. Even if poverty (however measured) did not exist, a government might, for moral or ideological reasons, still attempt to transfer resources between the rich and poor. However, it is not possible to find redistribution among the aims set for the social security system by any of the post-war governments.

The new project for social security

Passive and active aims

It is sometimes said of the Beveridge scheme of social insurance that it was essentially *passive*. By this it is meant that the post-war social security system was designed only to respond to the circumstances of people's lives and not to influence them. This reflected Beveridge's somewhat static view of society characterised by near full employment of a largely male workforce with the care of children undertaken by women within stable, two-parent, married households (Baldwin and

Falkingham, 1994; Hills *et al.*, 1994). So we can identify benefits which were used (or aimed) to prevent hardship and to maintain circumstances until the prior *status quo* of full-time employment would be resumed. This passive role is also identifiable in changes and innovations to the social security system in the 1960s and 1970s. Social and economic changes unanticipated by Beveridge (long-term unemployment, and the rise in lone parenthood, for example) have been met with corresponding changes to the benefit system (such as the introduction of higher long-term rates for unemployed claimants of social assistance, and the additional payments to lone parents in child benefit and income support). Equally, these policy innovations can be reversed as evidenced by the decision to remove the premium from lone parents making new claims after December 1987.

We can contrast this passive picture of social security with the more *active* use made of the benefit system in the last thirty years. In particular, we will look at how the social security system has been harnessed to the wider project of the 1980s' and 1990s' Conservative governments (and now Labour government) to construct a new economic and social order (Alcock, 1990).

Getting people into work

As we have seen, the origins of unemployment insurance lay in the desire to prevent people who cease working from descending quickly into poverty. It was seen as a form of temporary assistance that would only be required in the short term until people found new, full-time work. This passive role of unemployment benefit continued in the post-war Beveridge social security system. There was an assumption that the normal mechanisms of the labour market, assisted by a system of labour exchanges to bring unemployed worker and potential employers together, would ensure that the unemployed did not stay that way for very long. The phenomenon of long-term unemployment would, it was assumed, no longer be a feature of the British economy and society.

The structure of benefits for the unemployed reflected the assumptions of the post-war world. Qualification for benefit depended on a person being completely out of the workforce. You were either in full-time work and receiving a living wage or you were out of work and entitled to social security payments. Working and claiming benefits were seen largely as a contradiction in terms. The one exception was in the concession to people on social assistance benefits (i.e. the long-term unemployed) who were allowed to keep small amounts of money earned from work. This is the 'earnings disregard' which is still a feature of the income support scheme in the 1990s. Any amount earned above the disregard results in a pound-for-pound reduction in the amount of Income Support paid (the so-called 'poverty trap', Deacon and Bradshaw, 1983).

It has long been recognised that the benefit system for the long-term unemployed, while providing some level of financial protection, creates its own set of barriers to people trying to return to work. In addition to the 'poverty trap' mentioned above, many people were caught in the 'unemployment trap' in which a move to full-time work could mean an actual reduction in household income. In the 1980s a number of strongly held beliefs about unemployed people on benefits, part of the New Right ideology, had a profound effect on successive governments' approach to social security policy. One belief was that benefit levels were too generous, allowing claimants to have a reasonable standard of living without having to work. Another belief was that the benefit system was creating a dependency culture in which people looked first to the state to help them in times of difficulties rather than to their own efforts for other forms of support. From this powerful conjunction of the well-known negative effects of benefit structures and New Right ideology came a new role for social security – getting people into work, and helping them stay there (see, for example, Department of Social Security, 1995, 1998).

The concrete expression of this aim can be found in several changes and innovations in the social security system. Among these changes we can identify 'sticks' – disincentives to staying on benefit – and 'carrots' incentives to take work. The following are some examples: Family Credit[4] – a benefit which tops up low pay for families with dependent children; Disability Working Allowance – a benefit modelled on Family Credit which tops up low pay for disabled people; Jobseeker's Allowance[5] – the replacement for Unemployment Benefit and Income Support for the long-term unemployed, which reduces the amounts paid to unemployed claimants and imposes more conditions on them (about efforts made to find work); Earnings Top-Up[6] – another benefit modelled on Family Credit, for single people and childless couples; Incapacity Benefit – the replacement benefit for invalidity benefit for the long-term sick which has forced thousands of people back into the labour market who had previously been protected through the social security system.

Getting people into work can be seen as a marked shift in the aims of social security, away from the passive role of supporting people out of work to a more active role in encouraging people into work and discouraging them from relying solely on the benefit system for their income. Changing people's labour market behaviour is not the only way in which the social security system has become active. We now turn to attempts at changing people's behaviour in other ways.

Changing behaviour

One area of disagreement in studies of living on benefit concerns the quality of the lives of people on low income. For example, Bradshaw and Holmes, in a study of sixty-seven families living on benefit in Tyne and Wear, concluded that their lives were characterised by the 'unrelieved struggle to manage' (1989, p. 138). In contrast, Jordan *et al.* (1992), while not presenting a rosy picture of the material conditions of life on benefit or low income, depicted a community sharing and acting in much the same ways as the rest of society and constructing lives, albeit constrained, over which they had some control. From this we may conclude that life on benefit is not unchanging but that people can exercise some choices about their lives (see also Sainsbury *et al.*, 1996). However, those choices may not be to the liking of government, i.e. not accord with their view about how people should behave. Some examples, claimed by recent governments, might be parents (particularly mothers) who choose to live apart from their partners and live on a mixture of social security benefits, or young single unemployed people who choose to leave home and again live on benefits. It is not important for a discussion of aims whether one accepts that such views represent a social problem or even a reasonable picture of social reality. The point is that, if those with power over the social security system think this way, then social security can be used to discourage certain types of behaviour and encourage others. An aim of social security therefore becomes to change people's social behaviour.

Some recent examples of policy initiatives that have been directed at changing people's behaviour include the following: reducing the value of benefits for lone parents (including Income Support and Child Benefit) – with the intention of making life as a lone parent more difficult, and thereby discouraging relationship breakdown and encouraging existing lone parents to take work, live with relatives or repartner. Paying reduced benefits to single people under 25 years old – with the intention of discouraging unemployed young people from leaving the parental home and setting up an independent household. Restricting Housing Benefit payments to single people – again to discourage single people from living alone in rented accommodation. These measures can be seen as crude measures to reduce benefit expenditure and as ways of promoting (or enforcing) a model of the nuclear family put forward in recent times as the essential foundation of a stable and civilised society.

Conclusion

In this chapter we have reviewed what people have been trying to achieve through the social security system in the course of this century. It should be clear that it has not been a simple task to define what the aims of social security have been and are now. They have been many and varied, have changed and are changing. Aims can be stated in terms that are broad and vague (the 'vision' of social security) or can be defined in more precise terms that might serve as yardsticks by which the success or failure of social security policy and implementation can be evaluated. For the social security system as a whole we are more likely to be offered the former. It is more likely that we have a clearer idea of the aims of individual benefits (particularly when they are new) or of policy changes.

The aims of social security, as expressed by one political party or another, or by pressure groups and representative organisations, ultimately derive from some deeper system of beliefs about what constitutes the good society, about what should be constitute relationships between individual members of society and between citizens and the state (Hill, 1993). Such aims will extend beyond social security and find expression in almost every area of public policy such as finance and taxation policy, health, employment, social services or the environment. We should remember that social security is only one of many tools of policy at the disposal of governments in the pursuit of their wider aims.

In this chapter we have seen numerous examples of how since 1979 social security policies have been fashioned to support a wider set of aims for the transformation of social and economic life in this country. The tenets of the New Right philosophy of promoting the market economy, rolling back the frontiers of the state, and encouraging self-help, individual responsibility and economic independence are reflected in the aims set for the social security system over the same period. In the Departmental Report of the DSS for 1996 these were said to include 'focusing benefits on those who need them most, encouraging personal responsibility, and improving incentives to work and save' (DSS, 1996, p. 2). Two years later, and under a Labour government, the key phrase has become 'work for those who can, security for those who cannot'. It is possible that this list would look largely unfamiliar to the government of Lloyd George whose aim in establishing unemployment and sickness benefits was to protect vulnerable people from the threat of poverty and worse. However, a very different agenda (based on a different set of deep-seated beliefs) was being pursued then compared with now.

As we noted at the beginning of the chapter, we have chosen to present a discussion about aims, rather than, for example, what functions social security performs, in an attempt to show how complex, diverse and versatile social security can be as an instrument of policy. In any analysis of social security policy, therefore, simplistic notions that social security is there to relieve poverty or redistribute wealth should be avoided, and its inherently political nature and its possibilities for promoting or restricting welfare explicitly recognised.

Notes

1 For an interesting analysis of social security based on its social functions, see Spicker (1993) (particularly Chapter 8).
2 Both benefits were replaced in 1992 by Disability Living Allowance and a reformed Attendance Allowance.
3 National Assistance from 1948 to 1966, Supplementary Benefit from 1966 to 1988, and Income Support from 1988.
4 The forerunner of Family Credit, Family Income Supplement, was originally introduced in 1971 as a means of ameliorating the problem of poverty among families on low pay. It was not primarily seen as addressing the aim of getting people into work, but of trying to keep them in work (Brown, 1983; Corden and Craig, 1991). From October 1999 both Family Credit and Disability Working Allowance will be replaced by a system of payable tax credits.
5 Jobseeker's Allowance was introduced in October 1996.
6 Earnings Top-Up was introduced in October 1996 on an experimental basis in eight areas of the country for a period of three years.

References

Alcock, P. (1990) 'The end of the line for social security: the Thatcherite restructuring of welfare', *Critical Social Policy*, 30: 88–105.
Baldwin, S. and Falkingham, J. (eds) (1994) *Social Security and Social Change*, London: Harvester Wheatsheaf.
Beveridge, W. (1942) *Report on Social Insurance and Allied Services*, Cmnd 6404, London: HMSO.
Bradshaw, J. and Holmes, H. (1989) *Living on the Edge: A Study of Living Standards of Families Living on Benefit in Tyne and Wear*, London: Child Poverty Action Group.
Bradshaw, J. and Lynes, T. (1995) *Benefit Uprating Policy and Living Standards*, Social Policy Report No. 1, York: Social Policy Research Unit.

Brown, J. (1982) *Disability Income: Part I, Industrial Injuries*, London: Policy Studies Institute.

—— (1983) *Family Income Supplement*, London: Policy Studies Institute.

—— (1984) *Children in Social Security*, London: Policy Studies Institute.

Corden, A. and Craig, P. (1991) *Perceptions of Family Credit*, London: HMSO.

Deacon, A. and Bradshaw, J. (1983) *Reserved for the Poor*, Oxford: Basil Blackwell & Martin Robertson.

Department of Social Security (1995) *Social Security Departmental Report. The Government's Expenditure Plans 1995–96 to 1997–98*, London: HMSO.

—— (1996) *Social Security Departmental Report. The Government's Expenditure Plans 1996–97 to 1998–99*, London: HMSO.

—— (1998) *New Ambitions for our Country: A New Contract for Welfare*, Cm 3805, London: HMSO.

Fraser, D. (1973) *The Evolution of the British Welfare State*, London: Macmillan.

George, V. (1968) *Social Security; Beveridge and After*, London: Routledge and Kegan Paul.

Hall, P., Land, H., Parker, R. and Webb, A. (1975) *Change, Choice and Conflict in Social Policy*, London: Heinemann.

Hill, M. (1990) *Social Security Policy in Britain*, Aldershot: Edward Elgar.

—— (1993) *The Policy Process: A Reader*, London: Harvester Wheatsheaf.

Hills, J., Ditch, J. and Glennerster, H (eds) (1994) *Beveridge and Social Security*, Oxford: Oxford University Press.

Huby, M. and Dix, G. (1992) *Evaluating the Social Fund*, London: HMSO.

Jordan, B., James, S., Kay, H. and Redley, M. (1992) *Trapped in Poverty?*, London: Routledge.

Macnicol, J. (1980) *The Movement for Family Allowances 1918–45*, London: Heinemann.

Sainsbury, R., Hutton, S. and Ditch, J. (1996) *Changing Lives and the Role of Income Support*, DSS Research Report Series No. 45, London: HMSO.

Spicker, P. (1993) *Poverty and Social Security*, London: Routledge.

Thane, P. (1982) *The Foundations of the Welfare State*, London: Longman.

3 Development of social security

Pete Alcock

What role for social security policy?

Social security policy in Britain in the latter half of the twentieth century has been dominated by the structuring influence of the Beveridge Report on *Social Insurance and Allied Services* first published at the height of the Second World War in 1942. As we shall discuss shortly, Beveridge's report covered a wide range of policy issues and proposed a number of far-reaching and comprehensive welfare reforms; however, at the centre of Beveridge's concerns, and as the major focus of his planned reforms, was the need to remove the problem of poverty from British society – or 'want' as he called it. His hope and intention were that post-war social security policy would prevent the recurrence of poverty in Britain. If there are two central questions which this chapter should address, therefore, they are:

- how did social security policy seek to prevent poverty?, and
- did it succeed in this task?

Despite the important influence of Beveridge's work, both in setting the tone for debate about the role of social security and in shaping the development of future policy change, it would be wrong to see post-war British social security simply as a product of his vision of poverty prevention. Social security policy, like all other policy development, is produced not by visions but by the weight of historical circumstances and economic pressures and by the conflicts and compromises of political power. Beveridge's proposals themselves were, of course, a product of his recognition of the need to build on the strengths of the past and the present in seeking to shape the future (Harris, 1977); and as the proposals were implemented by the post-war Labour administration they became subject to the political pressure to meet a number of different needs and objectives (Lowe, 1994).

As J. Bradshaw has discussed in Chapter 1, the objectives of social security policy are not restricted to the prevention of poverty – even though Beveridge might have wished that they were. Indeed, even a focus on the prevention of poverty is far from controversial and can be contrasted with a focus on poverty relief. The former (prevention) is pro-active and the latter (relief) is reactive; and each leads to rather different models of social security protection (Alcock, 1997, Chapter 14). However, within Britain – and in all other welfare capitalist countries – social security policy pursues aims other than the prevention or relief of poverty, for instance, the redistribution of resources across the life cycle and the maintenance of past living standards. The changes in policy which have characterised the development of social security in Britain over the last fifty years are the product of the shifting demands of these and other priorities as well as of the role of current provisions in removing poverty; and judgements about the success or failure of policy development must take into account this broader context.

What a wider recognition of the differing policy goals of social security reveals, however, is the very diverse – and even contradictory – nature of the objectives for policy development. In meeting some goals, policies will inevitably miss others; and, overall, the balance sheet will inevitably be one of failures in some areas matched by successes in others. Over time, of course, and as policies change, this balance will shift; and it is the nature of this shift – and the policy decisions which lie behind it – which are the major focus of research and analysis of the development of social security policy. A key theme running through the book is on the problem of poverty, and so we shall concentrate here primarily upon the ways in which social security policy has responded to this problem (or has not!); but it should be remembered that it is only one issue amongst many.

Over a period of fifty years there have obviously been significant changes in political power and political priorities, and changes in underlying social circumstances and economic trends. There have also therefore been many changes to social security policy, both in terms of general structure and detailed benefit entitlement. We could not hope to cover all of these here, although there are specialist texts in the area which do seek to do this at least in part, notably Hill (1990) and Baldwin and Falkingham (1994). This chapter is a summary of major themes, and in particular of the influence of social science research on policy change. However, even coverage of change from such a perspective can easily slip into the form of a chronological list of significant events and political watersheds, and chronology provides only a limited understanding of policy development. Thus, while we will seek to trace the significant shifts in social security policy over time, we will also set these in the context of an ongoing analysis of their relationship with the major themes and concerns which underlay all policy debate and development.

When seen against these broader and ongoing concerns, the critical questions which we discuss below, the policy developments of the post-war period begin to take on a perspective of consistency alongside change. Although significant developments have been made and different agendas pursued, many of the important underlying issues have remained the same. What this reveals, of course, is that the problems facing social security policy are not altogether new, and that the means which might be adopted to respond to these have not departed radically from past practices. This may be a comforting, or a disturbing, conclusion to be reached for those who see in the lessons of the past the means for successful policy development in the future; but it is one which reminds us of the importance of the longer view in the assessment of policy reform.

Critical questions

The issues which have underlain social security policy throughout the post-war period in Britain provide us with a series of foci from which to analyse and assess policy changes. They have also been the basis for a range of theoretical and empirical research work seeking to analyse social security from these different standpoints, both over time and within particular political and policy conjunctures. They give rise to some critical questions which can be used to interrogate the historical development of policy change and to reveal the extent to which this change has responded to the goals which have been set for it.

The first set of questions concern the *people* for whom social security policy is intended – who are the intended recipients of benefits?; and do the benefits reach those groups in need of social security support? The second set of questions focus on the *principles* behind benefit provision – how are benefits delivered, and do the criteria for benefit entitlement lead to effective distribution of public support? The third set of questions address the *policies* behind the benefit scheme – what are the aims of policy development, and what are the structures adopted to meet those aims? Finally how, over time, have these three differing concerns interacted to shape social security policy; and how successful have they been in preventing poverty?

People

Social security policy is directed towards people. Individuals and groups are identified as needing, and deserving (or perhaps *not* deserving), financial support and benefits have been developed to provide entitlement to such support for defined categories of beneficiaries. Because of the principal concern of social security with the problem of poverty, the particular focus of this process is on the attempt to identify who is, or who might be, poor, with the aim of providing benefits either to anticipate or to relieve their poverty. While anyone may become poor, the risk of poverty is particularly associated with those in circumstances which are likely to lead to poverty – notably because of exclusion from the labour market or inadequate provision within it. What is more, as Rowntree's (1901, 1941) early research on poverty revealed, such exclusion is also linked to particular stages in the life cycle – notably childhood and old age.

Thus people are more likely to be poor at certain stages in their life cycle, in particular if they are unable to provide for themselves through wages in the labour market. Risk of poverty is particularly associated with childhood and old age, and with parenthood – especially where parents' resources are restricted by low wages or unemployment. As we shall see, it is these groups of people, and the need to provide support for them, which have dominated debate and research on social security policy in the post-war period in Britain.

Principles

The principles underlying benefit entitlement can also be reduced to a small number of major criteria, and policy debate has focused almost exclusively on these throughout the last fifty years. In Britain, and indeed in all other welfare capitalist countries, three major principles have been in competition within social security policy; and in practice all have played a significant, if fluctuating, role.

Universal entitlement is the simplest principle for determining access to social security support – payment is paid to all citizens in any particular group. The first of the modern social security benefits introduced in twentieth-century Britain, the 1908 old age pension, was initially a universal provision for all over-75s, although entitlement to pensions was later restricted by other criteria. Universal entitlement to benefit such as pensions does exist in some other countries, for instance in Scandinavia, today. In post-war Britain universal entitlement to benefits has been fairly limited; however, the reformed Child Benefit and the disability benefits introduced in the 1970s were universal, and, in the case of the former at least, have been successful in reaching virtually all who might be entitled to them.

The main theme underlying Beveridge's (1942) proposals for social security reform was the use of social *insurance* to determine entitlement to benefit protection. Insurance is a model for social security widely used on the continent, although, as we shall see, Beveridge's proposals were slightly different from most European systems (Hills *et al.*, 1994). Contributions towards a social security fund are made by those in employment and their employers; and entitlement to benefits during periods of interruption of employment are determined by past contribution record. Insurance thus provides support in return for contribution, appealing to a spirit of collective self-protection. However, it only provides protection at times of absence from the labour market, and it is only available to those who have made the requisite contributions in the past.

Because of the limitations of universal and insurance protection, therefore, post-war British social security provision has also included *means-tested* benefits. Means-testing is in fact the oldest principle in social security, going back to the ideals of the old Poor Law. Benefit support is only provided to those who can prove that they have no other adequate income or resources – in effect that they are poor – and this is established via a rigorous and intrusive test of their means. Means-tested benefits are also often referred to as *assistance*, and they have often attracted a stigma associated with the failure of recipients to provide for themselves. In practice, of course, assistance benefits provide a safety-net protecting those who 'fall through' other forms of support – but they can also be seen as a last resort to be relied on only when all else has failed (Eardley *et al.*, 1996).

Policy

Which of the different principles underlying benefit protection operate and to what extent are a product of the policy decisions taken by government; and different policy priorities have resulted in a shifting balance between these three principles over the post-war period in Britain. However, the policy options concerning social security extend beyond the criteria for benefit entitlement.

Governments must also decide on the extent of the state's role in providing social protection and the part to be played by private protection arranged by individuals themselves, or through their employers. Where state provision is provided, as J. Veit-Wilson discusses in Chapter

4, the level of protection needs to be set – how generous should benefits be? Then the maintenance of these levels must be secured, or changed – should benefits be increased in line with price inflation or with growth in overall wage levels? Throughout most of the post-war period wages levels have grown much faster than prices.

At a more general level still, governments need to take major policy decisions concerning the extent and direction of social and economic policy, and these will affect the way in which social security policy develops. Throughout all of the second half of the century governments have had to decide between seeking to extend the amount and scale of social protection or seeking to contain public expenditure and thus cut back on social spending. Furthermore, in terms of general economic development they have had to decide between redistribution of existing resources in order to ensure that those at the bottom have adequate support, and promotion of further production in order to increase the pool of resources for all.

The development of social security policy in Britain over the post-war period has been concerned continually with these key issues of people, principles and policies. Despite the considerable changes that have been made, the questions posed by the choices between them have remained at the centre of academic research and political debate. However, within these recurring themes we can identify some clear policy shifts. In particular, we can perhaps divide the post-war period up into three broad periods in which different policy contexts have been dominant. These are the legacy of Beveridge, the drift to selectivity, and the pursuit of privatisation and targeting.

The legacy of Beveridge

Beveridge's Report on social insurance, published to widespread acclaim in 1942, remains the most comprehensive and coherent review of the aims and means of social security policy produced in this country. Indeed, despite some claims to the contrary concerning the Fowler reviews of the 1980s (Green Paper, 1985), it is really the only attempt at an overall statement of policy direction. Harris's (1977) biography sets Beveridge's report in the context of his broader experience and interest in social and economic policy development. Together with the economic policy prescriptions of his colleague Keynes, Beveridge has been credited with the development within British policy of a particular kind of 'liberal collectivism' (Cutler *et al.*, 1986); and, shortly after the implementation of his social security plans, Marshall's (1950) reformulation of citizenship to incorporate social citizenship – the right of all citizens to basic social protection through the state – seemed to suggest that Beveridge had contributed to the creation of a new era of social solidarity after the Second World War (see Baldwin, 1994, pp. 37–55).

In fact, as Baldwin (1992) argues, important and wide-ranging though Beveridge's proposals were, they were the product of a careful balancing act between radical and comprehensive reform, and adaptation of past provision within a context of contradictory political pressures. Beveridge's legacy was one of both revolution and pragmatism.

Perhaps the most revolutionary aspect of Beveridge's Report was the context of policy reform in which he set it. Beveridge argued that his proposals for social insurance protection would be dependent for their effectiveness upon the introduction of Family Allowances to contribute towards the costs of child care and a National Health Service accessible to all, and upon the commitment by government to maintain full employment (for men at least). This assumed a significant shift in policy towards collectivism through the state, which was far from non-controversial in political circles (Addison, 1977). However, these changes were achieved, and they set the scene for Beveridge's contribution to the prevention of poverty through social citizenship.

Unlike previous social security provision Beveridge wanted the social insurance scheme to prevent poverty by anticipating the circumstances in which it might arise and by providing support through benefits in these circumstances. This required benefit support at a subsistence level, paid for by contributions which all would be obliged to pay. The scheme he proposed was collective, because all would pay and benefit; but it was based on a notion of insurance, so that all would feel entitled to state support – avoiding the stigma associated with previous means-tested provision. The subsistence benefits would be kept at a basic level, however, to avoid any competition with the wages which workers would receive and to ensure that the flat-rate contributions which all would pay would be sufficient to meet benefit costs. It was these basic principles of equal participation and equal treatment for all which gave Beveridge's scheme its appeal to social citizenship, and which made it so revolutionary.

In practice, however, none of these principles were all that new or radical. The insurance principle had, of course, been the major feature of previous social security protection both through the state and in the private sector. In a sense, all that Beveridge was proposing here was a merger of past protection into one single state scheme. Moreover, he did not envisage this comprehensive state provision replacing the role of private protection – indeed, one of the attractions of low state benefits paid for by flat-rate contributions was the scope they left for the better-off to supplement these with private insurance. Beveridge also relied upon continuity outside insurance in other respects; in particular his scheme assumed that family life would continue to characterised by the male breadwinner model, and so married women were largely excluded from direct protection within the scheme – although this did provoke some protest at the time (Abbot and Bompas, 1943; and see Baldwin and Falkingham, 1994).

Beveridge's insurance scheme was contested in other respects too. His proposals for social insurance were modelled in part on the kind of insurance protection developed in other European countries, and initi-ated in Germany in the nineteenth century by Bismarck. However, unlike continental social insurance which links benefit entitlement and benefit levels closely to individual contributions, Beveridge's scheme offered subsistence benefits to all in return for flat-rate benefits. The system thus operated from the start on a 'pay-as-you-go' basis, with contributions being used to meet current benefit needs; and this in a sense meant that contributions were little different from other forms of direct taxation. The Treasury were thus opposed to the separate contri-bution base, and Maynard Keynes and James Meade, acting as advisers on it, saw it at best as a temporary expedient to attract political support for the increased payments which in effect it would require (Glennerster, 1995, pp. 30–31).

It was because of Beveridge's belief in the popularity of the insurance base therefore that it came to dominate post-war social security policy, rather than any principled support for the model collectivism which it implied. Beveridge claimed that, 'The capacity and desire of British people to contribute for security are among the most certain and impressive social facts of today' (1942, p. 119). However, the setting of subsistence levels of benefit not only meant that the middle classes would be tempted into supplementing their state insurance protection with private support, it also meant that the insurance benefits which were paid might not be sufficient to meet the needs of all of those who were required to depend upon them.

The benefit levels in Beveridge's report had been based upon the primary poverty levels established by Rowntree in his research on poverty in the 1930s (1941). These were not generous levels, and they were reduced by the government when implementing the scheme. They also only included a basic contribution towards the cost of rent, although this too had been subject of controversy within government due to wide variety between rent levels throughout the country. The result of this was that benefit levels were lower in relation to average earnings than they had been in the 1930s (Glennerster, 1995, p. 90).

The low levels of benefit meant that at best Beveridge's post-war social security scheme must be regarded as a fairly minimal move towards social citizenship. However, the low levels of insurance benefits also had a more practical and ultimately, from the point of view of social security policy, more contradictory, consequence. Beveridge was aware that, despite the objectives of comprehensive coverage, not all in need would be guaranteed full protection from the social insurance scheme; thus he recommended the retention of means-tested provision through a scheme of National Assistance as a secondary – and demonstrably less desirable – safety net. His expectation was that, as the insurance scheme came to fruition, the need to depend upon assistance would gradually decline and fade away; but, because of the gaps and inadequacies of the insurance plan, this did not happen. When the assistance scheme was introduced there were one million people depending upon it, and by the 1960s this had grown by 50 per cent.

Thus, even when it was finally introduced by the post-war Labour government in 1948, Beveridge's plan for social security was in practice both limited and partial, and in particular had not resulted in the replacement of means-testing with insurance protection in the benefit system. However, when judged against Beveridge's primary aim – the elimination of want (poverty) – it success seemed to be fairly clear-cut. In 1951 a repeat of Rowntree's research on poverty in York revealed that the numbers of poor people had declined dramatically (Rowntree and Lavers, 1951).

People

The focus of Beveridge's plan for social security was on the provision of benefits for periods of interruption of employment. This was because the scheme was intended to be predicated upon the guarantee by government of full employment, although it also assumed that women could be provided for indirectly through the wages or benefits received by their husbands. As Glennerster (1995, p. 32) points out, however, this focus also appeared to be justified by Rowntree's (1901 and 1941) research on poverty, which revealed that, whilst low wages had been the major cause of poverty in the nineteenth century, by the 1930s this had been replaced by unemployment. If unemployment could be prevented, or provided for, poverty could be avoided.

Beveridge was also of course aware of Rowntree's remarks about the influence of life cycle changes on the risk of poverty. As well as focusing on interruption of employment through provision for unemployment and sickness, therefore, Beveridge's scheme also transferred resources across the life cycle by using insurance contributions to pay pensions to those who has retired from the labour market. Furthermore, the accompanying provision of Family Allowances, which Beveridge had argued for, provided some contribution towards the costs of child care (although not for the first child), thus ensuring that low wages would in effect be supplemented for poor (large) families. Family Allowances, old age pensions and short-term insurance benefits for interruption of employment should therefore have provided comprehensive coverage for all those at risk of poverty. However, by the end of the 1950s, ten years after the implementation of Beveridge's plan, evidence began to emerge that all these groups were not in practice being protected by the insurance scheme.

In part, because of the problem of rent costs, the insurance pension was not sufficient to meet the needs of all pensioners. Many thus had to claim National Assistance benefits too. Most of the one million assistance claimants in the 1950s were pensioners, and many more were probably entitled to claim but had not taken up their rights. Of course Beveridge's intention had been that the low basic pension would provide a floor on top of which individuals could invest in higher private or occupational pension protection. In the 1950s such occupational pensions (superannuation) had begun to develop; but they were often rather restrictive in scope, and they were divisive in that only a minority could benefit from them. Titmuss, Professor of Social Policy at the London School of Economics (LSE) and instrumental in the development of new research on social security policy in the post-war era, argued that they were creating 'two nations in retirement' (Titmuss, 1958, p. 74).

The Labour Party in opposition began to employ the services of Titmuss and some of his colleagues at the LSE to develop an alternative plan for pensions, which would ensure that all were provided with adequate protection within the state scheme. What they proposed was the extension of the principle of paying earnings-related contributions in return for earnings-related benefits, as used in most occupational provision, into the state pension scheme – in fact the adoption of a similar form of social insurance to that found in the Bismarck schemes on the Continent. However, it was to be another two decades before these ideas finally came to fruition – too late to achieve some of the aims their early academic supporters had hoped for them.

Academic research in the 1950s not only revealed that pensioners were not being protected from poverty by the Beveridge insurance plan as two of Titmuss's colleagues, Abel Smith and Townsend, also carried out research into the growing problem of family poverty. Using new methods (analysis of statistics such as the Family Expenditure Survey produced by the government itself) and adopting new definitions (the use of a relative measure of poverty drawn from the government's own benefit scales rather than the subsistence level set by Rowntree thirty years before), they published an influential research report which revealed that up to 2.25 million children were living in poor households (Abel Smith and Townsend, 1965).

The assumption which underlay Beveridge's proposals for social security was that unemployment, rather than old age or low family wages, was the major cause of poverty. By the 1950s, however, it was becoming clear that pensioners and families were still at significant risk of poverty and were not adequately protected by the insurance scheme. These groups, and the means of providing for them, were to dominate academic research and political debate over the ensuing three decades.

Principles

Beveridge's intention had always been that his plans for social insurance would provide comprehensive social security coverage for all; but the identification of pensioner and family poverty in the 1950s revealed major flaws in the insurance model. Family Allowances were universal, of course, not insurance benefits. However, their value had not kept pace with rising living standards in the 1950s with the result that they were not able to provide a sufficient supplement to the incomes of low wage families when compared with their entitlement under the insurance or means-tested schemes (Banting, 1979, p. 67). This universal support inevitably overlapped with other social security provision, and this relationship would require reform and readjustment as the scope of these schemes changed also.

Beveridge's plans for means-tested benefits was for a gradual demise. He shared the dislike of assistance which had become widespread during the 1930s, and he saw little problem in maintaining a secondary and stigmatising status for such benefits after the war, for this would only help to enhance the superior position of insurance protection. However, assistance benefits were designed to meet basic needs, including rent, whereas insurance benefits were not. When they were introduced, there was in practice little difference between the two scales (Bradshaw and Lynes, 1995, Chapter 2), and when the benefit levels were increased in the 1950s these limited relativities remained.

Therefore, over a million people were dependent upon means-tested support in the 1950s and, despite Beveridge's hopes for comprehensive insurance cover, since then this figure has grown inexorably – and ever more rapidly. In practice, the legacy of Beveridge was not comprehensive social insurance, but a mixed economy of universal, insurance and means-tested benefits. In the fifty or so years since his report was published, the development of social security has seen a change in the balance between these different principles as the policy decisions of government have gradually complicated the simple vision of prevention of poverty through collective contribution.

Policy

When the Beveridge Report was published in 1942 it was popularly acclaimed and warmly received by most shades of political opinion. Its vision of collective protection through social citizenship was also largely endorsed by the Labour government which was elected with a landslide majority at the end of the war. In the 1940s state intervention in the economy and state guarantees of social services were at the centre of policy development. In this context social insurance for social security was a natural legislative development; and most, though not all, of Beveridge's recommendations were translated into policy reform.

The social reforms of the 1940s were also largely supported by the Conservative governments of the 1950s, within the spirit of what some called *Butskellism* (see Addison, 1977, p. 275). The 1950s also saw a period of sustained and significant economic growth in Britain, and in the wider world economy, during which living standards rose. This meant that social policy provision could be maintained or extended without significant additions to either taxation or public borrowing; and during this period benefit levels were increased above the subsistence levels proposed by Beveridge and set by the government – although they barely kept pace with the more general rise in standards experienced by those in work (Bradshaw and Lynes, 1995).

For almost two decades after the war, therefore, social and economic policy appeared to be following an inexorable trend of growth and improvement, characterised by Macmillan's 1959 election slogan that Britain had 'never had it so good'. However, academic research had by then begun to challenge the success of social security preventing the recurrence of poverty in the country and to put pressure on government to change social policy in order to meet the continuing and growing needs of poor people. With the election to power in 1964 of a Labour Party, which had been influenced by this research while in opposition, there was hope that this might lead to new developments in social policy in the 1960s.

However, by this time there were influences other than academic research coming to bear on government policy-making. The Labour government of the 1960s inherited a period of economic growth that was gradually coming to an end. There was thus pressure to stimulate new economic development, and to set social policy changes against other priorities for the use of public resources. In such a context the policy commitment to social security through social insurance which had lain behind the implementation of the Beveridge plan began to come under pressure from alternative models of social protection, and social security development began to drift in another direction.

The drift to selectivity

The 1960s and 1970s were when, for the most part, the Labour Party was in government in Britain. Given Labour's original commitment to the implementation of the Beveridge plan and their sympathy towards arguments about the rediscovery of poverty within the affluent society of the 1950s voiced by academic critics such as Abel Smith and Townsend (1965), we might expect therefore that this period would have seen a renewed commitment to realising the comprehensive ideals of Beveridge's insurance proposals. Indeed, this is just what some academic critics and researchers argued should be the policy priority (Atkinson, 1969).

However, this is not what happened. Although reforms in the insurance scheme were made, they were piecemeal and much delayed; and overall the major effect of social security policy development was an increased reliance upon means-tested benefits and significant extension of their scope. By the end of the 1970s there were over five million people dependent upon the major assistance benefit (then called Supplementary Benefit): and, in a review of the operation of means-tested provision, the National Consumer Council (1976) counted forty-five different such benefits.

A major reason for the failure of governments in the 1960s to extend and improve on insurance provision was the deteriorating economic climate affecting the country. Over these two decades the British economy moved from boom to slump to (by the mid-1970s) deep recession. In such circumstances any improvements in social security policy would require strong political backing. However, despite the growing influence of academic research criticising the limitations of existing benefit provision, political support for social security reform was increasingly diverse and contradictory as new political priorities began to overtake the simplistic vision of the Beveridge plan.

The Labour government elected to power in 1964 and returned in 1966 with a larger majority had clear commitments to respond to the growing poverty identified amongst pensioners and low income families, and to reduce the growing dependency upon means-tested assistance benefits. However, as discussed below, political pressures and compromises reduced their ability to deliver on the initial two promises; and furthermore, rather than reducing the scale of means-testing, the government in effect extended and entrenched it.

In particular, this was achieved by the restructuring of the post-war National Assistance scheme into a new safety net provision renamed Supplementary Benefit. This gave stronger entitlement to benefits and an increased weekly rate, and it led to increased dependency upon the new benefit – although probably not as a result of increased take-up of benefit entitlement, as had been hoped by some in government (Atkinson, 1972, pp. 19–20). Increases in the costs of rent and of health service prescription charges in the 1960s also led to the development of new means-tested benefits to provide rebates from these for those on benefits or low incomes. This increased the extent of means-testing and set the scene for further such expansion in the following decade.

In his review of the social security policy of the 1964–70 Labour government for the Fabian Society, Atkinson (1972) concluded that, although there had been an overall increase in expenditure on benefits, this could largely be accounted for by increases in the numbers of claimants – notably pensioners and the unemployed – and that the introduction of Supplementary Benefits had not been a success. The overall conclusion of the Fabian Pamphlet in which he wrote (Townsend and Bosanquet, 1972) was that poverty had increased under Labour. This was not a popular message with many in the Party and it contributed to a growing tension between Labour and left academics; but it was evidence of a general trend identified by academic researchers which continued into the 1970s. The Fabian Society reached similar conclusions after the 1974–79 Labour government (Bosanquet and Townsend, 1980).

The economic pressures which faced the Conservative government of the early 1970s were greater than those on Labour in the 1960s, and also the Conservatives were less concerned about the growing use of means-tested benefits. Indeed, many Conservatives saw means-testing as a way of ensuring that those on low incomes could be protected from rising costs and that limited resources could be directed primarily to those most in need. In fact, these were arguments which had also begun to influence Labour politicians too in the 1960s (see Banting, 1979, Chapter 3). The Conservatives' major new means-tested benefit, Family Income Supplement (FIS), had been considered by Labour in the 1960s; and, in extending rent and rate rebates, and relief from prescription charges and other health service costs, the Conservatives were building on developments initiated in the 1960s.

In fact, the Conservative government of the early 1970s considered making a much more fundamental and comprehensive shift towards the use of means-tests, rather than insurance, as the central feature of social security provision through the replacement of all benefits with a system of 'tax credits', which would use the taxation system to focus support on all those with low incomes (Green Paper, 1972). This was never realised, although the principle of the merger of taxes and benefits as a replacement for current insurance and assistance social security benefits has remained as an ideal for some (Adam Smith Institute, 1984; Dilnot *et al.*, 1984).

Part of the reason for the failure of the Conservative government of the early 1970s to achieve its social policy reforms was the growing pressure of economic decline – with the numbers of unemployed, for instance, passing the one million mark. For the Labour government which followed later in the 1970s these pressures were even more acute; and in particular they led to a need to reduce the scope of public expenditure and thus to cut back on social policy goals, as exemplified in the White Papers on expenditure from 1975 onwards. Despite Labour's commitments to tackle poverty and reform social security, therefore, these pressures made the achievement of such promises extremely difficult.

In fact, in the context of the severe economic recession of the 1970s, Labour's record on social security reform was a relatively positive one. This period saw the culmination of the major reforms of pensions and family support and the development of new protection for the disabled. The government also began with a major increase in level of the basic pension and this was maintained by an uprating policy which linked pensions to both rising incomes and rising prices (whichever was the higher), and this was extended in practice to other benefits too (Piachaud, 1980, p. 174). Furthermore, short-term social insurance benefits were reformed to place them more firmly on an earnings-related basis – finally replacing completely the flat-rate principle of Beveridge and at the same time removing his unequal treatment of married women.

In the late 1970s therefore the increase in insurance expenditure was greater than the increase in the cost of means-tested benefits (Barr and

Coulter, 1990, pp. 285–289). Despite this, however, the numbers of people affected by means-testing continued to grow, in particular as a result of the larger numbers of people who were unemployed for long periods of time and thus were inadequately protected by insurance benefits, and because of Labour's continuation of the new means-tested benefits, such as FIS, introduced by the Conservatives. According to Piachaud (1980), therefore, the numbers on or near the margins of poverty remained high; and poor people remained at the centre of research and debate on social security policy.

People

Pressure for social security policy reform in the 1960s and 1970s came in part from the rediscovery of poverty by academic researchers and their argument that the Beveridge plan had failed in its major objective of preventing poverty. The rediscovery of poverty identified particular groups of people who remained inadequately protected by the insurance scheme, and much of the development of social security policy during this period focused on these groups. They were the elderly, the unemployed, low wage families and (later) the disabled.

It was the *elderly* who first of all were identified as receiving inadequate protection from flat-rate insurance benefits, as a result of which the better-off were supplementing these with private pensions and the worse-off were forced to rely on means-tests. Supported by academic researchers such as Titmuss, the Labour opposition in the 1950s had developed proposals to overcome this through the development of an earnings-related addition to the state insurance pension which would eventually benefit all – as happened in many continental countries; and in the meantime to introduce an increased income guarantee for all pensioners. However, the Labour government of the 1960s was unable to deliver these plans: the income guarantee was judged to be too expensive and was transformed instead into the restructuring of the National Assistance scheme, and the earnings-related pension proposals were introduced too late and were lost when Labour was removed from power in 1970.

The Conservative government of the 1970s were not committed to a full state earnings-related pension and wanted to encourage occupational pensions instead. They did, however, propose to introduce earnings-related contributions to support the basic state pension; but this too was frustrated when the Conservatives lost power in 1974.

Although the Labour government of the 1970s was quick to realise its commitment to raise the basic pension, it remained committed to the idea of extending the state scheme to include an earnings-related element. Labour was, however, wary of repeating the past reversals on pensions policy experienced by both themselves and the Conservatives. They thus sought tacit support from the Conservatives for a new state earnings-related pensions scheme (SERPS) which finally came into operation in 1978, and, as the price of Conservative support, operated in partnership with the private sector by permitting those with occupational protection to opt out of this element of the state scheme.

It had taken over twenty years to achieve this shift of pension policy towards the continental (Bismarckian) model, however; and it would be another twenty years before the full earnings-related additions which were accrued within it would begin to be paid. It thus did nothing to protect existing or prospective pensioners from poverty – hence the importance of the continued uprating of the basic flat-rate pension; but this was a principle on which Labour did not have Conservative support.

One of the most serious of the pressures on social policy resulting from the growing economic crisis of the 1960s and 1970s was the increase in the numbers of the *unemployed*. Beveridge's expectation was that government guarantees of full employment would mean that such interruptions from the labour market would be of limited duration and readily protectable through insurance. However, the low levels of insurance benefits meant that some unemployed claimants, especially those with children and high rents, had to supplement their insurance benefits with means-tested support. It was partly in order to avoid this, and also to cushion the blow of any increase in the numbers experiencing unemployment, that the Labour government of the 1960s – again following the continental model – introduced a earnings-related supplement to unemployment (and sickness) benefit for the first six months of entitlement.

The aim of the supplement was to take unemployed claimants off dependency upon means-tests. However, the six-month time period meant that the achievement of this became more and more difficult as periods of unemployment grew in length. Only around 20 per cent were receiving it in 1969 (Atkinson, 1972), and after that this proportion declined further. What is more it is arguable that the needs of unemployed claimants increase rather than decrease as the length of their unemployment extends. Yet the increase in basic benefits enjoyed by pensioners in the mid-1970s was not extended to the long-term unemployed; and by the end of the period the gap between the relatively generous protection afforded to pensioners when compared with the unemployed had become an important structural feature of social security policy.

It was *child poverty*, in particular the problems of families on low wages, which had been the most significant element of the rediscovery of poverty in the 1960s (Abel Smith and Townsend, 1965). It had even led to the establishment of a new and influential pressure group, the Child Poverty Action Group (CPAG), through which the research findings could be presented for political debate; and CPAG became a major vehicle for the dissemination of academic research throughout the last three decades of the century (McCarthy, 1986).

Child poverty in working families had grown in significance in the 1950s and 1960s because the Family Allowances intended to support child care had not kept pace with other rises in wages and benefits. Labour's commitment to respond to this problem in the 1960s therefore required them to address the question of the level of such family support. However, increasing the level of Family Allowances, which went to all families, was an expensive option at a time when resources were constrained. Labour politicians thus debated an alternative strategy of providing a means-tested supplement to low family wages which would focus support on those in most need (see Banting, 1979, Chapter 3).

This was an early example of the pressure to move towards selectivity which was to become more and more dominant in policy debate for the rest of the century. In fact it was resisted by Labour then by means of compromise measure under which the increase in allowances which was eventually agreed was 'clawed back' from those with reasonable incomes via a reduction in tax allowance. This link between taxes and benefits set the scene for the Conservatives' later consideration of a scheme for tax credits rather than benefits, however; and in any event they introduced a means-tested supplement to low family wages in FIS in 1971.

Labour continued the operation of FIS in the 1970s and, as we have seen, also extended other aspects of means-testing. However, they once again came under pressure from the CPAG and others to improve Family Allowances as an alternative means of tackling child poverty. This was achieved with the introduction of Child Benefit in 1977. Child Benefit was a universal payment for all children and it replaced both Family Allowances and child tax allowances for workers. In many ways it was a significant re-affirmation of this element of the Beveridge plan for poverty prevention, at a time of growing pressure for more means-testing of benefits, although its eventual emergence was a hard-fought battle against some of those in government who did not want to make such a commitment (Field, 1982).

People with disabilities had not constituted a recognised group among the poor at the time of the major post-war reforms of benefits; but by the 1970s both the increasing numbers of *disabled people* and the greater recognition of the specific needs which they experienced led to the development of new social security protections for them. Attendance Allowance was the first of these benefits introduced in 1971 to cover the costs of personal care. It was followed in 1974 by Non-Contributory Invalidity Pension, to cover living costs, and in 1976 by Mobility Allowance and by Invalid Care Allowance, a flat-rate payment for those providing care to disabled people.

None of these new disability benefits were paid at a very high rate, and in many cases they left disabled people and their carers still in poverty and dependent upon means-tested support. However, they were a recognition of the needs of a 'new' group social security beneficiaries, and they were paid on a universal basis – contributing to the continuing mix of benefits within the system.

Principles

By the end of the 1970s, therefore, the mix of benefit provision within social security had become ever more complex. Insurance benefits and universal benefits had been retained, and even expanded by Labour governments. However, means-tested benefits had grown significantly both in scale and scope. The Conservative government of the early 1970s had been the first post-war administration to pursue openly the extension of means-testing in preference to other benefits – notably through FIS. However, despite their manifesto commitments to reduce the role of means-testing, Labour had failed to do this, and in practice had themselves presided over a continuing growth in these.

Labour had seriously considered a benefit similar to FIS in the late 1960s, and in the 1970s they did not seek to repeal it. Furthermore in the mid-1970s they instituted an internal review of the major means-tested scheme, Supplementary Benefit, which in effect signalled their recognition that, since this could not be removed, it would have to be reformed. In fact the review, eventually published in 1978 (DHSS), was highly controversial, not least because of the injunction that no additional expenditure was to flow from it (see Donnison, 1982; Supplementary Benefits Commission, 1979). Labour did not act on the review; but in the early 1980s a new Conservative government did.

Policy

The policy climate of the 1960s and 1970s was not one which was very conducive to progressive social security reform. Economic problems went from bad to worse and as a result public expenditure was squeezed and then cut. In fact, despite this, throughout the period expenditure on social security grew both absolutely and relatively within social policy – even in the 1970s (see Barr and Coulter, 1990). In large part this was because the pressure of demand in the scheme was also growing, in particular due to growing numbers of pensioners and unemployed, and to the development of new benefit protections. Nevertheless, benefit rates were increased following inflation in either prices or earnings, whichever was the higher in any particular year (Bradshaw and Lynes, 1995); and policy commitments to major extensions of insurance and universal benefits were achieved – notably in the late 1970s. This was to be in stark contrast with the period following when the drift to selectivity became a headlong gallop towards targeting of resources within social security, and benefit rates began to be cut for the first time since the 1930s.

Privatisation and targeting

The election of the Conservative government under Margaret Thatcher in the 1980s has been seen as leading to a significant departure from the support for state welfare which had previously characterised the post-war period in Britain (Johnson, 1990), and to the rise to prominence within both academic and political circles of the 'New Right' (King, 1987). Quite how significant and far-reaching both the aims and the achievements of the Thatcher governments were in 'rolling back' state welfare, however, is certainly debatable; and there is no doubt that some of the wilder proposals emanating from the New Right were never seriously considered by government. At the same time, the Conservatives were faced with the continuing severity of economic recession, especially in the early 1980s, and thus the pressure on social policy reform remained firmly one of restraint.

In many ways the circumstances faced by the Conservatives in the 1980s were very similar to those which had confronted previous governments in the post-war period: the pressure to respond to the growing groups of the poor, and at the same time the need to restrict the expansion of public expenditure. However, at the same time, there were some major differences which characterised the Thatcherite response to these, and to a large extent the response of the Major governments which followed in the 1990s. These were the explicit rejection of the evidence of growing levels of poverty within the country and the commitment to pursue means-testing (or targeting, as it was now called) and private protection as more desirable forms of social security protection.

Conservative ministers of the 1980s were openly sceptical about the arguments that poverty was a product of economic dysfunction within modern industrial societies, suggesting instead that it was largely a product of individual inadequacy (Boyson, 1971; Joseph, 1972), and they also rejected the claims of academic researchers that relative poverty could be growing even in an affluent society (Moore, 1989). They thus rejected Beveridge's ideas of poverty prevention through insurance provision and sought instead to focus social security reform upon the relief of proven poverty. Important policy changes flowed from these new, and different, concerns; but as we shall see, although they altered the balance of provision within social security, they did not change the fundamental parameters.

In fact, Conservative reform of social security policy was an early political priority in the 1980s. They moved swiftly to implement the proposals emanating from Labour's review of Supplementary Benefits to set this major means-tested scheme on a consistent legislative basis. In the same year they sought to cut insurance benefits by breaking the links between pension uprating and wage increases – after this pensions only increased in line with price rises, reducing significantly their relative value (Bradshaw and Lynes, 1995, p. 10), by uprating short-term insurance benefits at below the rate of inflation – in practice a real cut, and by phasing out the earnings-related supplement to these benefits. These reforms resulted in a significant increase in the dependency upon means-tested provision.

This shift was carried further in the mid-1980s by the reform and extension of rent and rate rebates to become Housing Benefit, and by the tightening of eligibility criteria for short-term insurance benefits both through harsher tests of availability for work and tighter contribution requirements. Ironically, at the same time as these cuts on insurance benefit were taking place, the government was also increasing the amount of National Insurance Contributions (NICs) by raising the percentage of wages to be paid. This measure finally removed any traces of a direct relationship between contribution to insurance and entitlement to benefits. Of course, ever since Beveridge, contributions had only been used to meet current benefit liabilities; and in the 1980s when unemployment was rising rapidly, increased current costs were used as a justification for increased contributions levels at the same time as benefit levels were being cut.

The scope of insurance protection was also reduced in another way in the early 1980s, by the removal of entitlement to sickness benefit from the social security scheme and the replacement of this with a right to sickness pay from an employer. This was a measure of privatisation of social security provision which the government were to take further later, by extending the period of entitlement to sick pay and by transferring maternity provision also to employers. In fact, it did not do much to reduce the indirect public cost of provision for sickness (see Taylor-Gooby and Lakeman, 1988) but it was an important symbolic step, and it was followed more importantly in the late 1980s by the encouragement of more private and occupational provision for pension protection.

In addition to the reforms of benefit policy in the early 1980s, the government also introduced significant changes in the operation of benefit delivery. The individual pathology model of poverty championed by ministers such as Joseph and Boyson encouraged the belief in some government circles that many claimants might be inclined to accept too readily a continued reliance upon social security support – what came to be referred to as the creation of a 'dependency culture'; and even that some might be claiming benefits to which they were not really entitled. Fears thus developed about abuse and fraud within benefit provision. As research carried out in the 1970s had shown (Golding and Middleton, 1982), these were not new fears; but, fuelled by the media, the government of the 1980s gave them a much higher profile in policy debate and introduced a series of procedural measures within benefit offices to 'crack down' on the supposed levels of fraud and abuse – although frequently these were far from successful (see Franey, 1983; Smith, 1985).

The reforms of the early 1980s constituted a significant shift within social security policy; but they were largely piecemeal in nature, and, if they were a product of an overall strategy, they were not the product of coherent plan. In 1984, however, it looked as though this might change with the announcement by the then Secretary of State, Norman Fowler, of a series of reviews of social security policy. Fowler called these reviews 'the most substantial examination of the social security system since the Beveridge report forty years ago', and they took almost a year to complete. However, the reviews were in practice four separate examinations of different elements of the benefit system (Supplementary Benefits, Housing Benefit, children's benefits and pensions), and they ignored significant aspects of provision such as National Insurance. The review teams were also dominated by government ministers and government supporters, and they could hardly be characterised as an independent examination of problems and solutions.

In the end, the scale of the mid-1980s' reviews was far below that of Beveridge, and the reforms which they recommended (Green Paper, 1985) constituted largely a rationalisation of the existing complex means-tested provision in order to remove some of the anomalies and contradictions between different benefits and to reduce administrative costs. This primarily meant a restructuring and paring back of Supplementary Benefit (now to be renamed Income Support), and the alignment of entitlement to this with Housing Benefit and an extended version of FIS (to be called Family Credit) to create a single entitlement regime for these major means-tested benefits and to reduce some of the worse problems of the poverty trap and take-up levels which had been associated with them (see Deacon and Bradshaw, 1983, Chapters 7 and 8). These administrative changes proved to be rather complex to intro-duce themselves, however, and, although legislation was passed to implement the reforms in 1986, the new measures did not come into force until 1988 – after the Conservatives had won a third election victory.

There was thus no new overall vision behind the Fowler reviews, and no genuinely radical proposals for reform in them – except the plan to repeal the 1975 state earnings-related pension scheme and to replace it with new inducements for people to take out private pension protec-tion. Of course it had been Labour's hope that the earnings-related state scheme would attract the support of the Conservatives, and they saw its potential disappearance now as a major blow. However, they were not the only ones. The private pensions industry was not interested in the removal of a state scheme which they could not hope to replace, and the representatives of both sides of industry also made it clear that they would not welcome such a drastic extension of privatisation. Thus in the ensuing legislation the plan to replace SERPS was dropped and instead cuts were made in entitlement to it which would not take effect until the early twenty-first century – far enough to remove debate about these to another political agenda.

The 1988 social security reforms thus revealed the limitations which faced the Thatcherite plans for privatisation and targeting. Although they made many minor changes to entitlement and to levels of benefit, they did not fundamentally alter the structure of benefit provision. Means-tested benefits were reformed but their basic structure was retained, insurance benefits were largely untouched except for the future cuts in SERPS, and even universal Child Benefit was retained –

although in the late 1980s its value was allowed to fall against inflation by failure to upgrade it regularly.

Nevertheless, 1988 was in many ways the high-water mark of Thatcherite reform. Changes were continued after that time, notably the removal of 16- to 19-year-olds from any benefit protection and a continuing tightening of unemployment benefit entitlement; but they were not of major policy significance. What is more in the 1990s, when Major replaced Thatcher as Prime Minister, some changes were even reversed – for instance Child Benefit upgrading was restored. Although in the mid-1990s the restrictions on the scope of insurance benefits continued with the introduction of a less generous long term sickness benefit (Incapacity Benefit), and the replacement of Unemployment Benefit with a Jobseeker's Allowance, a flat-rate benefit payable only for six months and subject to stringent tests of job search.

In the late 1980s and early 1990s the emphasis of reform also shifted to some extent from changes in benefit entitlement to changes in benefit delivery. The introduction in new technology was by this time in any event transforming the procedures for the delivery of benefit payments. These technological changes were not, however, without their teething problems, however, and these problems were compounded by a range of other measures introduced to restructure the administration of social security in order to meet government commitments to devolution and privatisation. Most notably significant areas of administration were passed from the DSS to independent agencies, such as the Benefits Agency and the Contributions Agency; and some other aspects were subject to 'market testing' in preparation for transfer to private operators.

For many Conservatives on the New Right the primary hope for social security policy in the 1980s and 1990s had probably been that the introduction of reforms should see an end to the inexorable growth in expenditure on benefits. Yet against this measure, even more than all others, the record was largely one of failure, for expenditure continued to expand – reaching around £90 billion a year in the mid-1990s. Of course this was in large part a product of an increase in the numbers of beneficiaries rather than any increase in the levels of benefit (Barr and Coulter, 1990, p. 292); and, as research on the 1988 changes revealed, these reforms largely operated to redistribute resources between categories of claimants rather than generate any long-term savings (Evans *et al.*, 1994). Thus in broader policy terms, as we shall see below, increasing expenditure was in a sense only another manifestation of the same problem – the inability to reduce the dependency of people upon state support.

This is a problem which was also inherited in 1997 by the New

Labour government elected on 1 May. The new government sought to tackle dependency head-on with an extended emphasis upon the encouragement of long-term benefit claimants to enter the paid labour market – generally referred to as a plan for 'welfare to work'. This included as a new programme of employment and training, financed under a 'windfall tax' on the privatised utilities (called the 'New Deal'), and a restructuring of means-tested support for low wages through a Working Families Tax Credit to make low paid work more financially attractive. The new government thus took on board many of the policy priorities of the previous Conservative administrations, although they were also aware of the need for a longer-term strategic approach to the problem of welfare dependency, plans for which were outlined in a Green Paper released in 1998 – to be implemented early in the twenty-first century.

People

The reforms of the 1980s, therefore, had failed to bring about a radical overhaul of social security. They had also failed to halt the growing levels of poverty and inequality which had become widespread within the country by this time. In the early 1990s the Joseph Rowntree Foundation commissioned a series of research projects to examine trends in poverty and equality over the last few decades of the century – almost one hundred years after Rowntree's (1901) original research on poverty in York, which had set the scene for much policy debate in the earlier part of the century. The research was wide-ranging and covered income trends both within and outside the labour market. However, the overall conclusions, summarised by Barclay (1995) and Hills (1995), revealed a depressing consistency – levels of poverty had been growing in Britain in the latter part of the twentieth century (and especially in the 1980s), and the gap between the rich and the poor had been getting greater. If we are to judge the success of social security policy primarily by its ability to prevent poverty, as we suggested at the beginning of this chapter, then these were damning findings.

   The Rowntree research was not alone, however. The government's own figures on household incomes revealed that the incomes of the bottom 10 per cent of the population had declined in real terms by 17 per cent over the 1980s and early 1990s, while the incomes of the average had risen by around a third (DSS, 1995). Evidence also revealed that the groups of people at risk of poverty were also growing and changing. The elderly poor had grown in absolute terms, but they no longer constituted the majority of those in poverty; and new groups such as the long-term unemployed, families on low wages, lone parents and disabled people and their carers had now appeared in large numbers (Oppenheim and Harker, 1996).

Academic researchers, particularly those working on the European anti-poverty programmes, began to identify these emerging groups of poor people with the development of a 'new poor' in the 1990s (Room *et al.*, 1990). What in particular characterises the new poor is their exclusion from insurance protection and their dependency upon means-tested benefits; and this was certainly the case in Britain as a result of policy changes of the 1980s. However, other more pejorative assessment suggested that this exclusion was more far-reaching and was evidence that such people now constituted a new class (the 'underclass') with different social circumstances and different social values from the rest of society (Murray, 1990 and 1994; and see Morris, 1994).

Debate about the development of an underclass in Britain in the 1990s has now been widely joined (see Smith, 1992), and is beyond the scope of this chapter. However, in its focus on the groups of people most likely to be at risk of poverty it is really no different from those debates over classes of beneficiaries which were taking place at the time of the Beveridge Report and after. The people who are poor in the 1990s may be in somewhat different circumstances from those who were poor in the 1940s – although not in fact significantly so; and the debate over how social security policy should respond to that poverty faces a similar range of options.

Principles

The principles which underlay the response of the social security system to the problem of poverty have remained remarkably constant throughout the post-war period. It is the balance between these different principles which has been the subject of change.

It is debatable whether Beveridge's plan for social insurance could ever have provided comprehensive protection from poverty for all, and in practice it has certainly not done so. Thus, throughout the post-war period, the scope of insurance benefits has been in decline in policy terms as more and more people have become dependent upon a wider range of means-tested support, and, as in the 1980s, protection was transferred to the private sector. As a result, the numbers dependent upon the major assistance benefit, Income Support, in the early 1990s had reached ten million.

It is true that in the 1980s and 1990s in particular these changes have been the result of a deliberate pursuit by government of a policy of privatisation and targeting. But it should also be remembered that private pension protection developed in the 1950s and that most of the major schemes for targeting had their roots in the 1960s and 1970s. Furthermore, they have both been taken up in the New Labour agenda on welfare reform. Yet, at the same time the retention of SERPS, albeit in a reduced form, has revealed the continuing need, and support, for blanket insurance protection within social security. Pensions remain the largest expenditure item in the social security budget; and in the 1990s universal benefits for child care and disability needs have also been retained and even expanded. Means-testing may have become a more important – even a central – feature of British social security protection; but its has not become the dominant one.

Policy

During the early years of the post-war period social security policy was dominated by the aim of preventing poverty through comprehensive benefit provision within a growing economy – the vision of Beveridge. By the 1990s policy priorities had shifted dramatically to the need to contain, and ideally to reduce, expenditure on benefits in the context of continuing economic decline and restructuring, and consistently high levels of unemployment and benefit dependency, graphically spelt out in 1993 in a Department of Social Security discussion paper outlining the fears behind *The Growth of Social Security*. Thus, while the policy agenda of the 1940s focused on the problem of how to expand social security, the policy agenda of the 1990s has focused on the problem of how to contain it.

As a result of this, the concern of academic research with the growing levels of poverty and inequality in the country must now be set against the priority of government to limit rather than to extend their responsibility for responding to this. Abel Smith and Towsend's (1965) early pioneering research on poverty in post-war Britain received widespread political debate, fuelled by the new political pressure brought to bear by the Child Poverty Action Group. Nevertheless, it was ten years before the Child Benefit for which the campaigners calling was finally introduced.

In the 1990s there is much more academic research, and a much expanded CPAG, again pointing out that poverty exists – and, indeed, is getting worse. However, in the political arena the message is a more muted one, as other priorities dominate debate. As we have seen in this chapter, bringing about change in social security policy is a slow and complex process; and, in their 1998 Green Paper on welfare reform, the

New Labour government outlined a strategy for reform through to the year 2020. Perhaps twenty years may not in reality be too long to expect to wait for future reforms to flow from current research and debate on poverty – unless of course you are one of those who are poor.

References

Abbot, E. and Bompas, K. (1943) *The Woman Citizen and Social Security*, Bompas.

Abel Smith, B. and Townsend, P. (1965) *The Poor and the Poorest*, London: G. Bell & Sons.

Adam Smith Institute (1984) *Omega Report: Social Security Policy*, London: ASI.

Addison, P. (1977) *The Road to 1945: British Politics and the Second World War*, London: Quartet.

Alcock, P. (1997) *Understanding Poverty*, 2nd edition, London: Basingstoke: Macmillan.

Atkinson, A. (1969) *Poverty in Britain and the Reform of Social Security*, London: Cambridge University Press.

—— (1972) 'Inequality and social security', in P. Townsend and N. Bosanquet (eds) *Labour and Inequality*, London: Fabian Society.

Baldwin, P. (1994) 'Beveridge in the *Longue Durée*', in J. Hills, J. Ditch and H. Glennerster (eds) *Beveridge and Social Security: An International Perspective*, Oxford: Clarendon Press.

Baldwin, S. and Falkingham, J. (eds) (1994) *Social Security and Social Change: New Challenges to the Beveridge Model*, Hemel Hempstead: Harvester Wheatsheaf.

Banting, P. (1979) *Poverty, Politics and Policy: Britain in the 1960s*, London and Basingstoke: Macmillan.

Barclay, P. (1995) *Joseph Rowntree Foundation Inquiry into Income and Wealth, Volume 1*, York: JR Foundation.

Barr, N. and Coulter, F. (1990) 'Social Security: solution or problem?', in J. Hills (ed.) *The State of Welfare: The Welfare State in Britain since 1974*, Oxford: Clarendon Press.

Beveridge, W. (1942) *Report on Social Insurance and Allied Services*, Cmd 6404, London: HMSO.

Bosanquet, N. and Townsend, P. (eds) (1980) *Labour and Equality: A Fabian Study of Labour in Power, 1974–79*, London: Heinemann.

Boyson, R. (1971) *Down with the Poor*, Churchill.

Bradshaw, J. and Lynes, T. (1995) *Benefit Uprating Policy and Living Standards*, York: SPRU, University of York.

Cutler, T., Williams, K. and Williams, J. (1986) *Keynes, Beveridge and Beyond*, London: Routledge and Kegan Paul

Deacon, A. and Bradshaw, J. (1983) *Reserved for the Poor: The Means-Test in British Social Policy*, Oxford: Basil Blackwell and Martin Robertson.

Department of Health and Social Security (1978) *Social Assistance: A Review of the Supplementary Benefits Scheme in Britain*, London: HMSO.

Department of Social Security (1993) *The Growth of Social Security*, London: HMSO.

—— (1995) *Households Below Average Income: A Statistical Analysis*, London: HMSO.

Dilnot, A., Kay, J. and Morris, C. (1984) *The Reform of Social Security*, Oxford: Clarendon Press.

Donnison, D. (1982) *The Politics of Poverty*, Martin Robertson.

Eardley, T., Bradshaw, J., Ditch, J., Gough, I. and Whiteford, P. (1996) *Social Assistance in OECD Countries: Synthesis Report*, Department of Social Security, Research Report No 46, London: HMSO.

Evans, M., Piachaud, D. and Sutherland, H. (1994) *Designed for the Poor – Poorer by Design: The Effects of the 1988 Social Security Act on Family Incomes*, London: LSE STICERD, WSP/105.

Field, F. (1982) *Poverty and Politics: The Inside Story of the CPAG's Campaigns in the 1970s*, London: Heinemann.

Franey, R. (1983) *Poor Law: The Mass Arrest of Homeless Claimants in Oxford*, CHAR/CPAG/CDC/NAPO/NCCL.

Glennerster, H. (1995) *British Social Policy Since 1945*, Oxford: Blackwell.

Golding, P. and Middleton, S. (1982) *Images of Welfare: Press and Public Attitudes to Welfare*, Oxford: Basil Blackwell and Martin Robertson.

Green Paper (1972) *Proposals for a Tax Credit System*, Cmnd. 5116, London: HMSO.

—— (1985) *Reform of Social Security, Volumes 1, 2 and 3*, Cmnd 9517–9, London: HMSO.

—— (1998) *New Ambitions for Our Country: A New Contract for Welfare*, Cm 3805, London: HMSO.

Harris, J. (1977) *William Beveridge: A Biography*, Oxford: Oxford University Press.

Hill, M. (1990) *Social Security Policy in Britain*, Aldershot: Edward Elgar.

Hills, J. (1995) *Joseph Rowntree Foundation Inquiry into Income and Wealth, Volume 2*, York: JR Foundation.

Hills, J., Ditch, J. and Glennerster, H. (eds) (1994) *Beveridge and Social Security: an International Perspective*, Oxford: Clarendon Press.

Johnson, N. (1990) *Reconstructing the Welfare State: A Decade of Change 1980–1990*, Hemel Hempstead: Harvester Wheatsheaf.

Joseph, K. (1972) speech to the Preschool Playgroups Association, 29 June.

King, D. (1987) *The New Right: Politics, Markets and Citizenship*, Basingstoke: Macmillan.

Lowe, R. (1994) *The Welfare State in Britain Since 1945*, Basingstoke: Macmillan.

McCarthy, M. (1986) *Campaigning for the Poor: CPAG and the Politics of Welfare*, London: Croom Helm.

Marshall, T. H. (1950) *Citizenship and Social Class*, London: Cambridge University Press.

Moore, J. (1989) 'The end of the line for poverty', speech to Greater London Area CPC, 11 May.

Morris, L. (1994) *Dangerous Classes: The Underclass and Social Citizenship*, London: Routledge.

Murray, C. (1990) *The Emerging British Underclass*, London: Institute of Economic Affairs.

—— (1994) *Underclass: The Crisis Deepens*, London: Institute of Economic Affairs.

National Consumer Council (1976) *Means Tested Benefits*, London: NCC.

Oppenheim, C. and Harker, L. (1996) *Poverty: the Facts, Revised and Updated*, 3rd edition, London: CPAG.

Piachaud, D. (1980) 'Social security', in N. Bosanquet and P. Townsend (eds) *Labour and Equality: A Fabian Study of Labour in Power, 1974–79*, London: Heinemann.

Room, G. *et al.* (1990) *'New Poverty' in the European Community*, London: Macmillan.

Rowntree, B. S. (1901) *Poverty: A Study of Town Life*, London: Longmans.

—— (1941) *Poverty and Progress: A Second Social Survey of York*, London: Longmans.

Rowntree, B. S. and Lavers, G. (1951) *Poverty and the Welfare State*, London: Longmans.

Smith, D. (ed.) (1992) *Understanding the Underclass*, London: Policy Studies Institute.

Smith, R. (1985) 'Who's fiddling? Fraud and abuse', in S. Ward (ed.) *DHSS in Crisis: Social Security under Pressure and under Review*, London: CPAG.

Supplementary Benefits Commission (1979) *Response of the Supplementary Benefits Commission to 'Social Assistance: A Review of the Supplementary Benefits Scheme in Britain'*, London: HMSO.

Taylor-Gooby, P. and Lakeman, S. (1988) 'Back to the future: Statutory Sick Pay, citizenship and social class', *Journal of Social Policy* 17 (1): pp. 23–39.

Titmuss, R. (1958) 'The social divisions of welfare: some reflections on the search for equity', in R. Titmuss, *Essays on 'the Welfare State'*, London: Allen and Unwin.

Townsend, P. and Bosanquet, N. (eds) (1972) *Labour and Inequality*, London: Fabian Society.

4 Poverty and the adequacy of social security

John Veit-Wilson

What is meant by 'adequacy', and in particular the adequacy of social security? Why does adequacy matter and to whom does it matter? This chapter aims to introduce the issues surrounding the concept of adequacy in income maintenance systems and their relationship to ideas and measures of levels of living and of poverty. It addresses four key questions about adequacy – for what? for how long? for whom? who says so? – and considers if UK social security is adequate.

In this chapter, the term 'social security' will be taken to include categorical, contributory and means-tested forms of state income maintenance cash benefits. Where means-tested systems of benefits and exemptions are meant, the general term 'social assistance' is used, or the specific national name. The scope of income maintenance by the state, in its wider and narrower senses, is discussed in this chapter. Unless otherwise stated, the concept of adequacy is discussed in terms of material and social resources people need in order to achieve specified standards and qualities of living in their societies.

Why does adequacy matter?

Adequacy matters for both moral and functional reasons. Some people believe that no member of modern societies[1] ought to suffer from enforced deprivation of what society defines as required for decency and dignity. The adequacy of earnings and social security are issues of self-interest for everyone who experiences the precariousness of employment. Some people have always suffered from this insecurity; increasing numbers are experiencing it as the labour markets are restructured, yet it is widely seen as functional to the workings of productive labour markets and economies. Inadequacy of resources also matters to everyone who encounters or copes with the consequences of social exclusion, irrespective if their motive is compassion or fear. In modern society, poverty and its consequences affect everyone in some way, indirectly if not directly.

A great deal has been written about what it means to be poor and deprived in the UK and elsewhere, offering evidence that social security incomes or low earnings have long been inadequate for a participatory lifestyle (Kempson, 1996). Some of the statistics of inequality in money incomes or control over resources through time are discussed elsewhere in this book (see Chapter 1). But this vast body of evidence of poor lives still tells us nothing about what resources would be just enough to prevent them. Similarly, the statistics of inequalities cannot tell us anything about the adequacy or inadequacy of those unequal incomes. To find out what adequate social security would be, we need independent measures of the range of resources required to enable people to take a minimally decent and dignified part in social life, and to know what part social security plays among those resources. This chapter is therefore not about the evidence of poverty and inequality but about these adequacy issues alone.

What is the income maintenance system?

Security in the total experience of living is provided by many factors, intangible as well as material, collective as well as personal, by stocks of resources as well as by flows of income, in kind as well as in cash. Within all modern societies the flow of cash income forms a valued part of the total 'power over resources through time'[2] which individuals, families or households need in order to achieve and secure the socially recognised and approved levels of living. It implies status and gives self-esteem as well as giving access to opportunities for choices and exchange into valued goods, services and experiences.[3] Social security is only a residual part of income maintenance as a whole, which governments may provide when the normal parts of the system fail to do their job properly. The income maintenance system includes everything which affects the flows and stocks of money resources people have with which to meet their needs. This system can be defined widely, to include factors like health and housing, education and job opportunities, or more narrowly to focus on all kinds and sources of incomes, savings and taxes.

The level of a household's disposable income has usually been influenced by the interaction of a large number of these factors, as well as by its own needs. Therefore one cannot read off the adequacy of a total household income from the level of cash benefits alone. It may be affected by government action over any of these other areas, singly or in combination. Minimum wages and tax thresholds are equally important parts of the whole picture. Governments have power (even if they choose not to use it) to take the resources needed for participation partly or wholly out of the market system and distribute them in other ways, such as on the basis of individual need or collective benefit. Governments make choices about managing the different parts of the income maintenance system, and different social or income groups vary widely in the value of the benefits they receive in different ways – what is known as 'the social division of welfare' (Titmuss, 1958 and a large subsequent literature). How one judges the growth in inequality and poverty in the UK in the 1980s (Hills, 1995) depends on one's values. It was seen as desirable by people who welcome social inequality and define poverty in terms of static material standards (Moore, 1989), but unacceptable by egalitarians and those who see poverty as dynamic. Values and ideologies set the standards; politics writes the agendas; social science examines the results.

Values and ideologies

In such a value-laden subject, the underlying approach must be set out first. In every society there are conventional assumptions and beliefs which affect social behaviour, including the beliefs about the ways in which power should be exercised by some on behalf of themselves and others. One of the most important values refers to people themselves: either all people matter, or some matter less than others. In the end, we have to decide what matters most: each human being, or something else such as 'society', 'the nation', 'the economy' or 'the laws of history'. This is often expressed in religious or ideological terms but it does not need to be.

Other values relevant to this discussion are those of solidarity or of individualism (members of society should care about each other because of their common membership, or individuals should care only for themselves and their dependants). Note how argument also takes place about the elasticity of such values, about the boundaries of such societies and who a person's dependants are (or even 'who is my neighbour?'). The answers to such value questions influence our judgements about the strategies used by governments to ensure adequacy of resources for all in society or only for some. This is the realm of political ideologies.

The abstract term 'adequacy' has many meanings; this chapter discusses only those which concern sufficient resources to support a certain minimally-acceptable level of living. What that level of living is depends on the society and time in which it is lived. That social context also defines the resources which are needed to take part in that society and be recognised in it as having decency and dignity. The terms 'decency' and 'dignity' describe and summarise how people need to be treated and what they need to experience in order to achieve the qualities of participation in and belonging to their societies, reflecting the value that they matter.

The context of adequacy

What are the income maintenance contexts in which the concept of adequacy arises? There are at least three distinct aspects:

1   What people need for a decent level of living in modern industrial society, and what is meant by deprivation and poverty when people's resources are insufficient to meet socially defined needs. The boundaries between adequate and inadequate resources are often described as poverty lines.
2   How these questions are perceived by governments and whether they affect government policies. The standards governments use for assessing the adequacy of their income maintenance policies have been called Governmental Minimum Income Standards (MIS) (Veit-Wilson, 1998).
3   What role in meeting needs is played by the current government's income maintenance policies as a whole and social security in particular. Adequacy of social security affects how people dependent on it can achieve the decent level of living mentioned above.

Each of these is a large subject in itself and aspects have been discussed elsewhere in this book. Since they are often confused with each other, the box shows some distinctions (extracted from Veit-Wilson, 1998, p. 8).

Endless trouble is caused by trying to force poverty lines into politically credible forms. The term 'poverty line' should certainly not be used for both scientific and political measures indistinguishably. The discussion of the adequacy of social security is strictly a matter of examining the MIS used by governments and of their benefit scale levels, including the means tests for the remission of charges. It may refer to the findings of social science research about poverty lines but MIS are not poverty lines and are themselves often based on other government considerations and political objectives.

'Poverty lines' are best described as the income levels or bands which are statistically found most closely to the boundaries between:

1   high probability of correlation between high rates of complex socially defined deprivations and low incomes; and
2   low probability of correlation between incomes and deprivations.

Poverty lines are *scientific* measures of the minimum incomes individuals and households are discovered to need in order to take part in the society in which they live and to avoid what is defined as deprivation and exclusion in that society.

There are broadly two kinds:

1   *empirical poverty lines* based on statistical survey evidence
    a   showing the minimum income levels at which people *in fact are able and do* take part decently in society and avoid deprivation, or
    b   showing what the *population itself* reports would on average be just sufficient to 'make ends meet'.
2   *prescriptive poverty lines* based on experts' calculations of the minimum income which ought to be sufficient for minimally decent participation as socially defined *if* used according to the budgeted prescriptions based on (empirical) evidence of prevailing adequate living patterns.

Scientific research into poverty boundaries shows what that society's standards of adequacy are, irrespective of their political implications. The judgement about adequacy, the minimally acceptable real level of living, comes from social science evidence of society's standards and *not* from considerations of political viability or cost.

Governmental Minimum Income Standards are *political* criteria of the adequacy of income levels for some minimum real level of living (for a given period or indefinitely, of some section or all of the population) embodied in or symbolised by a formal administrative instrument or other construct.

Government MIS are often called 'official poverty lines', but the standards used are based on political decisions and not scientific findings (although the MIS could make use of them). The standard of adequacy of MIS is primarily a *political* reflection of that government's values, ideology and electoral considerations.

Social security and social assistance benefits are based on *political* decisions about how much the government is willing to pay to people in certain categories. Not all the recipients of social security are categorised as poor, nor is its aim necessarily to provide a sufficient income to combat poverty. The aim may be to help people maintain their previous levels of living, or support their own efforts to get out of poverty. Though by definition designed for the poor, the actual levels of social assistance may be demonstrably inadequate to meet minimum income needs for social participation.

Social security and social assistance benefits levels are based on MIS in some countries. Social assistance benefit levels are sometimes called 'official poverty lines' but this confuses the political decisions on standards and benefits with the scientific evidence of income needs.

The standard of adequacy of social security is primarily a political consideration of feasibility and cost.

Among the considerations which European Union governments may take into account is the recommendations of the European Commission on the importance of setting standards of adequacy. The European Commission has in recent years taken initiatives to encourage member states to protect not only their workers but also those who have been unable to enter the labour market or who have left it (Guibentif and Bouget, 1997). It asked member states to consider the minimal adequacy of their income maintenance provisions, recognising 'the basic right of a person to sufficient resources and social assistance to live in a manner compatible with human dignity' and 'to organise the implementation of this right' by 'fixing the amount of resources considered sufficient to cover essential needs with regard to respect for human dignity, taking account of living standards and price levels in the Member State concerned, for different types and sizes of households' (EC, 1992).

Elsewhere, the EC uses such phrases as a level of living 'worthy of a human being', or the ability to 'appear in public without shame', or to 'take part in the life of the community', as well as defining the poor as 'persons whose resources (material, cultural and social) are so limited as to exclude them from the minimum acceptable way of life in the Member State in which they live'. In Europe, therefore, the 'adequacy' of social security must therefore mean benefits large enough to enable people to live 'in a manner compatible with human dignity'. A minimally adequate level of living or decent way of life must be one which respects human worth and dignity and does not lead to people being ashamed or excluded.

There is thus no simple or even single answer to the question of what an adequate level of social security benefit might be. The concept of adequacy itself can be explained only if we first specify our objectives in context. Whichever word we use – adequacy, sufficiency, enough, necessities, needs, minimum – can be understood only if we explicitly state for what, for whom, and according to whom (Dubnoff, 1985). If the objective is a particular level of living, then one must ask not only about its contents but also for how long, the duration for which it is to be adequate. The questions about perspectives – for whom the level of living is adequate and who says that it is – are often forgotten, but they are absolutely inseparable from the question of contents and duration. What is enough for you may be too little or too much for someone else; it may be enough for a short time but not for long; what you think about the question may differ from other people's views. But the questions need not remain at this general and subjective level: collective agreement is possible and can be implemented by governments.

The next section of the chapter addresses the general issues raised by the four questions about adequacy, drawing examples from other countries beside the UK. The final section briefly reviews the basis of social security in the UK, showing that adequacy issues have never so far played a part in government thinking.

Adequacy for what?

Before the question of 'adequacy for what' one must establish what people require in order to live in society. This is the much-argued question of human needs.

Human needs

The concept of human needs covers a wide field. Just as with the word 'adequacy', needs can be discussed only in terms of the question 'needed for what?' Here is a brief and all-embracing definition of human needs based on a clear objective:

'Human needs' means the full range of intangible and material resources that are required over time to achieve the production, maintenance and reproduction of the fully autonomous, fully participating adult human in the particular society to which he or she belongs. The most basic needs every human has are the intangibles of having a society to be a recognised member of, and meaningful and supportive relationships throughout life within it. Material resources may support the physical organism but it is the full range of social and psychological resources which are required for the experience of humanity.[4] This statement about human needs is not a matter of dogmatic belief. If it is contested, the argument must be in terms of what is discoverable about all human societies and the resources required for societies to exist and for humans to flourish in them. It must not be about what someone elsewhere thinks is necessary or redundant among those resources. The important distinction between the social scientific approach of discovering what is needed, and people's ordinary approach of prescribing what ought to be needed (from some subjective point of view) is often overlooked, and this confusion between the empirical and the normative has seriously hampered the proper discussion of the subject of needs and adequacy.

The list of all the tangible and intangible resources required over a life span or even longer to enable a human being to become and remain a fully autonomous and participating adult member of his or her specified society would be a long and detailed one. It would be made even more complex if one includes what is required to provide and maintain the spatial and economic context in which that society continues and reproduces itself. The various human societies exist under widely differing geographical and economic conditions and have always each defined in different ways what they mean by full participation. Abstract definitions of needs are therefore no guide to what is required in specific social contexts. This is what is meant by saying that human needs are always relative to the society in which they are expressed.[5] The specific resources required to meet needs inevitably vary by social context, time and possibility. Where the resources are lacking or are withheld, then the needs may not be met and the individual or group can be described as deprived in terms of that society and its definitions of needs.[6]

Perspectives on poverty measures

The idea of poverty has taken many forms over the past century in which definitions and operational measures have been developed, and some of the issues have been discussed in earlier chapters. Many of the arguments concerned artificially low measures such as 'primary poverty' or 'minimum subsistence'. These approaches were asocial, that is, they were not concerned with ideas of adequacy for human life as it is lived in real society (Veit-Wilson, 1986, 1992). Asocial measures like these were instead constructed in order to make debating points about intolerably low incomes (for instance, Rowntree, 1901) or to justify setting social security levels below low wage rates (for instance, Beveridge, 1942). People devise poverty measures for a variety of different and conflicting purposes (Veit-Wilson, 1998, pp. 38–40) and anyone can set up such artificial measures; the question is, what are they set up for and what relation do they have to the realities of social life?

To address the purpose of how to identify the poor in social terms and distinguish them from the non-poor (for instance, in order to count them or study the causes of their poverty) social scientists have used a variety of methods to try to define and discover the boundaries of deprived levels of living, the condition of poverty based on inadequate resources, from which the poor suffer. Townsend (1954; 1962; 1979) was among the first to stress that because the standards by which an adequate level of living is defined in practice (even if not in the abstract) must inevitably come from society itself, poverty can logically be defined only in terms of lack of the minimum level of resources required to take part in society according to that society's own standards. Prescriptions based on other societies or other standards cannot function as criteria of poverty as such, whatever other purposes they may fulfil.

Since money functions as a virtually universal resource, one approach to assessing the adequacy of incomes is to see how far they enable people to acquire socially defined necessities (Gordon and Pantazis, 1997; Mack and Lansley, 1985; Townsend, 1979, 1993). Social surveys discover scientifically what the majority of people in that society and time take to be the social necessities which no one should be without. These are in fact only a small selection of all the resources needed for an adequate level of living, but they act as key indicators of actual or potential deprivation. The surveys also discover at what income levels people on average are deprived of one or more of these socially defined necessities. These approaches may confine themselves to identifying as deprivation indicators just a few of the key resources and experiences which people acquire by spending their own disposable incomes (Mack and Lansley, 1985), or they may include wider ranges of resources including access to intangibles and resources provided collectively or at any rate not out of personal disposable incomes (Townsend, 1979). For instance, one may not be 'poor' if one lacks the resource of social acceptability, but one may be unable to participate fully in society and thus be deprived in many ways.

Such an approach does not necessarily find a single cash threshold or draw a hard 'poverty line' between the poor and the non-poor. Mack and Lansley's national surveys in 1983 and 1990 found that most households across the income scale could claim to suffer enforced deprivation of one or two social necessities, but that three or more deprivations were clearly correlated with lower income. The boundary was thus a band of income, above which there was no probable correlation between income level and a low number of deprivations, and below which there was a high risk of correlation between greater deprivation and lower income. Similarly, Townsend and his colleagues' survey work in London (in 1985–86) suggested that there were broad thresholds of income below which there were higher clusterings of socially defined multiple deprivations (Townsend and Gordon, 1993).

Some social scientists have approached the question of discovering social measures of poverty more narrowly in terms of the material resources, particularly personal disposable money incomes, needed for an adequate level of living. Among the approaches adopted from this perspective are those which ask samples of the population to estimate the minimum income levels they need 'to get along' or 'to make ends meet'. From this point of view, poverty has been defined as having an income below one of these levels, or such that the family or household can only make ends meet 'with some difficulty' (Van den Bosch, 1993). If one assumes that social values and conditions are similar, then different expenditure patterns can also be indicators of adequate or deprived levels of living. Is a household of given composition spending enough to meet its nutritional or cultural needs adequately according to the standards of its society?

Each of these approaches raises many questions. Some are technical, concerned with the survey or statistical methods used. But behind them lies the larger issue of the choice of necessities and of standards. Each of these approaches has abstracted just a few of the human needs from the enormous list which could be composed. The deprivation indicator approach takes key resources and discovers the income levels at which people are deprived of them, assuming that the remaining multiplicity of resources would also be acquired or are irrelevant to the question posed. The attitudinal approach to minimally adequate income levels also ignores the many other material and social resources, taking them as being outside the frame of the question for those purposes.

The specific context of our question about adequacy is therefore the sphere within which people do or do not have enough personal disposable income to meet those of their socially defined needs which in this society they expect to meet by spending money. We are not looking at those requirements which are not bought, important though they may be. The next contextual issue is then the scope of the system within which people are enabled to acquire enough money.

Many resources, material, social and psychological, are required in combination to enable people to take part decently in society and to achieve dignity in their experience. The adequacy of people's control over each of these resources can be measured in terms of its ability to achieve the objective. But social security is primarily about governments transferring cash resources, and, in that context, adequacy of social security means benefits which provide at least the minimum income claimants require in their specific circumstances to meet the goal of enabling them to take a decent part in society according to the relevant prevailing social standards (adequate level), and to have the benefit administered in a way which enhances their dignity (adequate tone).

But a simple assertion about a participation standard of adequacy for incomes still leaves several questions unanswered: for instance, does the minimally adequate amount needed vary by the length of time one has to live on it? Is there and ought there to be more than one standard of participation, and if so, how should it differ between people and in cost? From whose perspective are these different standards defensible? We turn now to examine these further questions.

Adequacy for how long?

What period of time do we have in mind when we talk about the adequacy of resources to meet specified needs? The time-scale in which needs can be identified may vary enormously. At the shortest it can mean immediate satisfaction of an individual's urgent unmet needs. At the other extreme, if the objective is the continuity of human societies and the maintenance of the integrity of the earth's environment, it will be longer than any individual life-span.

Time-scale

How can we tell which time-scale is relevant to identifying needs? Some approaches have assumed that the key identificatory issue is urgency. Maslow's much-quoted hierarchy of five levels of need (1943, p. 395) ranged from non-postponable physiological needs to long-term self-actualising 'higher' needs, each level coming into consciousness as the preceding level was satisfied. Originally devised prescriptively in the context of planning employment incentives, Maslow's approach has little value in reflecting how people themselves rank their needs. Doyal and Gough among others point out (1991, pp. 35–36) that people pursuing dangerous sports appear to rank self-actualisation higher than physiological safety, and in any case what motivates people may not be a good guide to a description or ranking of their needs.

In reality, the question of time-scale often arises in the context of our assumptions about what the reasons are for needs being unmet, and who should be responsible for meeting them. For instance, if we see someone is thirsty or hungry, ill-educated or homeless, we may assume that the instant need is for a drink of water, some food, schooling or a home. The immediate problems of ensuring adequate provision to meet the needs of, for example, refugees and other migrants, force longer-term considerations out of the picture.[7] But if we ask how the need is to be met and who is to meet it, then we have to look at the availability of the resources required and who is responsible for providing them. Enormous capital investment in infrastructures and staff are needed for the supply of food or water, houses or schools. The time-scale may be reckoned in years and the costs will be far beyond the capacity of any individual to pay. Thus the interpretation of an individual's immediate needs presupposes that in his or her society there is a prior long-term provision which has been made by collective activity, whether capitalist or cooperative – and it is this which sets the context for the definition of individual needs over time.

The normal way of calculating what to charge for such long-term costs of provision is to add up everything taken into account[8] and divide the result between the users. But when are we users of, for example, schools or hospitals? We benefit from the education of others as well as ourselves, especially between generations, just as we do from knowing hospitals are there even when we are not using them. Thus the adequacy of the direct resources needed, or of the money people may need to pay for them through taxes or charges, cannot be measured in simplistic terms of who is using the resources just now. The same issues apply to individual needs for resources over a long period. An important example of the issue of time-scale in assessing the adequacy of social security arises when we consider the level of means-tested social assistance benefits in the UK and other countries (for example, Income Support since 1988).

One of the most important issues has been, are the weekly or monthly minimum benefit levels meant to be enough only for what is consumed during those periods? Or should they also cover some saving for durables which are not bought as frequently but which need replacing from time to time, 'lumpy purchases' such as bedding and furniture or the larger clothing items?[9]

From the UK's original social assistance scheme (Unemployment Assistance (UA) introduced in 1935) onwards,[10] the administrators have been either ambivalent or downright mendacious about whether the benefits were meant only to meet immediate subsistence needs or be adequate also for savings to replace durables. The planners of the UA scheme explicitly excluded everything from their calculations of minimum benefit needs except weekly expenditure on food, clothing, fuel/hygiene and rent, but within weeks of the introduction of the scheme, claimants asking for help to buy other items were being told by officials that the benefits were enough 'for all normal needs' (Veit-Wilson, 1989, p. 84). What they meant was not that benefits were enough for all the normal needs of families participating fully according to the prevailing social standards, but that the low-paid working-class families had to live on similar levels normally, even if they could not participate. To these officials, 'normality' therefore meant an inadequate level of living over time and not participation in normal society.

Similarly, a government departmental survey in 1964–65 found that National Assistance officials were making similar statements to claimants, either out of ignorance or a misplaced desire to save departmental funds at the cost of claimants' rights (Veit-Wilson, 1999, pp. 141–144). While the Supplementary Benefit scheme from 1980 to 1988 covered exceptional needs very explicitly as additions to the weekly scales, the Income Support scheme has implied they are generally included, since the Social Fund which may cover their cost usually does so in the form of loans to be repaid out of the weekly benefit. The inability of low-income families to repay such loans is commonly used by officials as a reason for not granting them (Huby and Dix, 1992).

The problem is similar in other countries. For instance, countries such as Germany and Sweden have used studies of minimum levels of living over a year or more as the basis of their national recommendations to local authorities for social assistance scales.[11] But the local authorities, who administer social assistance in these countries, often decide to cut out the cash sums which are meant to cover savings for the repair or replacement of household goods periodically. Their reason is that the spells of dependence on social assistance are merely temporary; claimants will not be dependent long enough to need to repair or replace items, and if they do they must make a separate application. But they may justify higher benefit scales for people who are expected to be long-term claimants, such as the disabled or elderly. In this respect, their argument is similar to that which justified the Long-term Addition to Supplementary Benefit in the UK from 1966 to 1988. We might want to argue about such differences, for instance, if we believe that the principle of equity requires that even short-term claimants should receive enough social assistance to be able to save for their longer-term needs if other citizens are expected to have enough discretionary income to do so. The ability to save is an aspect of taking part in normal society.

The adequacy of a person's disposable income (from sources such as social security) over a period of time can be assessed only in terms of what a person whose dignity is recognised would need in order to continue to take a minimally decent part in society over similar short or long periods of time.

This argument about the adequacy of income levels for shorter or longer periods, depending on what has to be covered and what conventional standards are, often gets mixed up with two different arguments. One argument confuses the minimum amount of money which people need (in order to achieve the socially defined adequate level of living over time) with the amount of money governments are willing to pay in social security and social assistance benefits for shorter or longer periods. The first of these is a question which can be answered only by the findings of social science research; it is not the same as the political matter of setting benefit rates, perhaps to be paid from taxation.

The second argument confuses the issue of duration adequacy with the question of how different social groups experience the adequacy of social security over different periods of time. This is really a question of 'adequacy for whom?' rather than of 'how long?' and is discussed next.

Adequacy for whom?

Whose needs are we talking about? When benefit levels are under discussion, it is commonplace that some publics and policy-makers in the UK have used the stereotype that social security or assistance is only for 'them' not 'us' and then only for short periods of time. But the assumption that society can be divided into 'we the people and they the poor' (as Sargent Shriver put it during the US 'War on Poverty' in the 1960s) is not supported by the evidence. Most people in modern industrial societies share similar values and aspirations, and what are sometimes described as (sub)cultures of poverty are not chosen (and certainly not genetic) but arise from material deprivations and social isolation (Brown and Madge, 1982; Valentine, 1968). The distinction between those currently poor or not poor is valid only in the very short term. So many more people pass through periods of poverty, or of dependence on social assistance benefits, than are poor just now, that in the longer term the better distinction for the majority of the population may be between those currently poor and those at risk of poverty at some future point in time. When currently non-poor people consider the adequacy of social security, the thought that they themselves may have to live on it in the future can radically change their perception of its adequacy.

Precariousness

Precariousness of adequate income has always been a problem for some sections of the population in industrial society, as Rowntree (1901) pointed out in his graphic description of the poverty cycle. This assumed constant low household earnings but fluctuating numbers dependent on them. But fluctuation also applied to the demand for working-class labour, and this has been increasingly experienced during the past few decades, at least in the UK, by what were previously thought of as the economically secure middle classes. Changes in the labour market such as the increasing insecurity of even middle-class occupations, in the patterns of occupational careers and in employment conditions, and also in family construction and break-up, have meant that wider population groups across the social class spectrum are at risk of experiencing periods of income inadequacy according to their own current social expectations and standards (Falkingham and Hills, 1995; Walker with Ashworth, 1994).

The greater the level of material affluence enjoyed over time, the more that a person may have built up existing commitments based on that level of cultural expectations. A major example in the UK is mortgages to buy houses. What a person sees as an adequate level of social security in unemployment or family separation to continue to meet these commitments may then vary according to the degree of subjective relative deprivation (Runciman, 1972) they apply to the judgement. Different social class experiences of enjoying courtesy, deference and accuracy from, for instance, bank employees may also lead to varying judgements of the psychological adequacy of the 'tone' of social security, the way in which the system is administered. An example is the contrast between the public acquiescence in the inadequate tone of Income Support but reaction against similar shortcomings in the Child Support Agency.

Compensation

A similar position arises when we consider those aspects of social security which aim to provide compensation for diswelfares, for example, the consequences of illnesses or injuries. What is judged to be an adequate level will depend on a variety of assumptions about the style and level of living which the individual has experienced previously and should now be provided. Allowing for additional expenses, is the level of living on social security benefits to be similar to that which other claimant groups experience, or should it vary; and if so, how and why? Examples of stratified practice and its inconsistent justifications in the UK are clear when we consider the differences in the current treatment of injury cases in which legal judgments can extract sums large enough for lifetime maintenance, generally from insurance firms, and those in which the 'causal agents' of the diswelfare cannot be identified and sued, leaving the damaged individual dependant on Invalidity Benefit or its successor, Incapacity Benefit.

Stratification

In each social context we have to ask two questions about standards. First, is there only one reference level of living to measure participation against, or conventional lifestyle to pursue, or more than one? Second, and separately, ought this to give rise to stratified standards in measuring the adequacy of social security?

This is no place for a clever 'postmodernist' argument about the impossibility of ranking the acceptability of a variety of forms of freely chosen lifestyles. In spite of the adoption of unconventional lifestyles by some (mainly younger) people, most people are still traditional in rejecting lifestyles associated with poverty if they have the choice. For millions of people the issue is brutal and immediate: they are deprived of what their society defines as social necessities, and they cannot take a dignified part in ordinary society without them. Only when these unmet needs are satisfied might they, too, consider the question of their own choices of lifestyle. This reveals that the relevant question is whether people have the resources with which to make their own choices between differing lifestyles, so that they can take part in conventional or eccentric lifestyle as they wish and are not forced into a low-status lifestyle without choice. Adequacy of resources therefore means having enough with which to exercise freedom of choice about participation, not suffering social exclusion enforced by inadequate resources. Within modern society, individual freedom of choice (in many even if not all areas of life) is of course an aspect of autonomy, an important psychological resource absolutely required for even minimal social participation.

At the national level in modern industrial states, the question of this stratification of expected standards varies considerably. Research into governmental minimum income standards (which may not be the same as the level of actual social security or other income maintenance benefits) shows wide variations in the degree of social stratification of standards (Veit-Wilson, 1998, pp. 79–82). At one extreme lie the Nordic countries where the prevailing assumption is that the minimum social assistance standards must be 'reasonable'.[12] The governmental organisations which devise the measures take this to mean 'for all citizens', by no means just for the poor. Indeed, the entire focus of social concern in Nordic countries until very recently has been on society's average level of living; the question of poverty was disregarded. At the other extreme lie countries like France, Germany and USA, where the prevailing assumption is that the standards need only be adequate for the low-paid working-class's level of living; no one would defend them as good enough for the middle class. In between, there are countries like Australia and the Netherlands where the adequacy standards are related to measures of minimum wages, in other words for low-paid workers, but where the conventional lifestyle is relatively undifferentiated in class terms and the minimum standards are relatively high and would probably be minimally acceptable to average citizens.[13]

Ethnicity

The question of adequacy for what in these class-stratified contexts is then seen as adequacy of what for whom, since the 'what' is assumed to vary by social class lifestyle. In countries with an ethnic mix, the question of class may be subsumed under other questions of cultural difference in lifestyle. The minimally adequate resources required to meet needs will then be defined in different ways. For instance, although the USA is an enormous ethnic mix, the prevailing assumptions about adequate lifestyles are remarkably homogeneous (consumerist, based on conventional European ideas of the family as the basic unit for the distribution of resources). By contrast, in Aotearoa/New Zealand's much smaller population there are three very different ethnic groups, Maori, Pakeha (European) and Pacific Islander. Each has its distinct patterns of familial sharing, and therefore a single concept of adequacy of social security is very problematic, since neither the units within which sharing takes place, nor the resources to be shared, are the same (Waldegrave and Frater, 1996).

To summarise, the question of adequacy for whom in income maintenance must be answered in terms of how far any stratification of culture, lifestyles and levels of living in a country are tolerated or even prescribed, and how far and why these differences are then supported by the government's social security system. This is not the same question as that of implementing equal citizenship rights. The Germans and French would probably argue that their Constitutions entitle all citizens to equal rights, for instance in Germany to a level of social assistance 'worthy of a human' (*menschenwürdig*). At the same time, they see that humans are differentially placed in material terms in society and believe that human worth and belonging to society are compatible with wide ranges of material inequalities. Similar claims were made in European pre-industrial feudal society. The issue can be tested empirically: do not only the majority of the population but even the recipients of the lowest level of social security experience that the benefits enable them to pursue a minimally decent level of living as defined in that society, and maintain their dignity as members of it?

The adequacy of social security must also be tested in terms of who it is for. In a stratified society, a variety of benefit levels may be justified in terms of protecting differentially placed people against subjective relative deprivation. Each previous level of living will have its own assessment of adequacy. But the key issue for poverty is *whether the lowest benefits are minimally adequate for everyone in that society according to its prevailing standards of decency and dignity.*

To answer the question therefore requires us to examine the values about human worth and the power to impose them which are held in different societies. Egalitarians will argue with the proponents of traditional feudal views (who hold that that hierarchically unequal but integrated organic communities are possible) about the adequacy of single or multiple standards for social security benefits. But the key issue for poverty is whether the lowest level of benefits would be recognised by all as providing decency and dignity. Again, this is not the same issue as that of political ideologies about the role of the state using its powers one way or another; the humanistic values may cut across the simplistic left-right divide about how to implement them.[14] This leads us to the fourth question, adequate according to whom?

Adequate according to whom?

Whose perspectives? Poor or non-poor? Who knows best what people's needs are? For most things, we assume we ourselves are the best judges of our own needs: what are essential necessities and what are luxuries we could do without if we had to. We know what we want to eat, but when there is a technical question of nutritional needs then we turn to the experts. But they are there to advise us, not to decide on our behalf what we should eat. And we certainly do not want other people telling us how to live.

So why are we so keen to do it to other people? If we look at the way the poor are treated by governments in the UK, we see that they are not trusted to know their own interests best. Richer people have always used their power to define poorer people's needs, but their self-interested prescriptions have no validity as guides to what the majority of ordinary people in society think are necessities for participatory adequacy. Both science and consistency suggest that the only reliable way of finding out what are socially defined necessities and the income levels at which they are available is to carry out social research. If people are to be valued, their opinions must be made to count in the definition of what they want to participate in. What are subjective views at the individual level become an objective social fact at the level of whole populations.[15]

But those who are poor rarely get to play any part in the discussion of the adequacy of their resources; the talking is generally conducted by the non-poor in terms of what they are prepared to pay the poor. Various social actors may take part in this argument. For instance, there are those who are poor now, and those, many more, who may at some point in their lives become so if the income maintenance system is not improved. There are those who are not poor and who fear having to share their resources with the poor, for instance by taxation or (in insurance risk sharing) by having to pay higher premiums to cover other people's higher risks. There are also governments at national and local levels with many competing claims on their resources. And there are the social and other scientists studying the other actors and sometimes getting into the act themselves, as experts advising governments and other groups on questions of adequacy for some purpose.

Asking the poor alone what they need will, however, give an incomplete picture of what the non-poor define as required for participation. The people who live in deprived situations may be so used to their unmet needs and so lacking in resources to meet them that they have realistically adjusted their expectations and life-styles downwards.[16] Better placed people must not then assume that the poor have freely chosen this low level of living or constrained lifestyle. Nor must they confuse the consequence, the way in which people cope with inadequate resources, with the cause: their poverty. Some people keep up appearances and starve themselves; others try to eat, clothe, warm and entertain their families and neglect appearances.

Whose perspectives? Expertise

The question of who is talking about who else's needs applies to every aspect of life. It runs from the most concrete examples of how much housing space and amenities people should have, or variety in the food they eat and stock of clothing they buy, or how much to spend on taking part in social life, to the most intangible examples of how much respect and politeness people expect in their relationships and exchanges with others.

Those who control technical knowledge, the experts, often play a role in setting such standards. To take three of thousands of examples, a government committee advised on the minimum adequacy standards to which local authority housing should be built to enable people to live decent lives in it.[17] Other expert committees advise government on the nutritional content of food and on health aspects of lifestyle. In the commercial sector, experts on marketing advise companies on attractive modes of selling their products by being courteous and considerate to customers, and this too affects the styles of behaviour which people come to expect in their dealings with public suppliers of services.[18] But the technical knowledge and advice itself and the contexts in which they can be offered are not uncontestable. Decent housing may be unaffordable; diets can be chosen only from what the commercial markets offer; tax cuts diminish resources available for public sector personal services. The 'experts' are people bringing their own social presuppositions into the question. The questions they are asked to advise on are only those which the current government considers important. The experts retained by governments are those with views they like; other equally expert views may be ignored.

Expertise which conforms to the natural science ideal model of openness, replicability and testability, can help to discover and expose the issues surrounding the adequacy of any standard. But opaque dogma, even from officially recognised experts, may have no more validity in establishing defensible adequacy standards than any other subjective opinion on its own. The poverty academics may try to develop tools which have the integrity of the social sciences; the governmental people are instead concerned with setting standards which symbolise their social values, their ideological beliefs and aspirations, and their specific policy objectives – and which have political credibility.[19] MIS reflect power and ideology, not necessarily scientific integrity.

Package deal thinking

When people suggest that others in the same society have generally different human needs, that is social stratification. People who are unequally placed in society often have taken-for-granted ideas that when they talk about minimum standards to meet needs, they mean good enough for the less well-placed. Anything more might be 'too expensive', although if the standards were for themselves they would be 'not good enough' or worth paying more for. But we must not deny the demonstrable existence of people's socially defined needs just because someone else does not want to share the costs of meeting them. To do so is an example of 'package deal thinking' (Fox, 1979) when testable facts get muddled up with values and beliefs about what ought to be, and both of them with the strategies to be pursued to achieve it.[20] Each of these should be considered separately.

Government objectives

Whose government is it anyway? What responsibilities should it have to intervene in the workings of markets and other mechanisms for distributing power over resources through time, in the interests of those who lack resources for adequate participation? Who should ensure that the costs of ensuring adequacy for all are paid, and that the costs of diswelfares are not allowed to lie where they fall?[21] This enormous field of argument is relevant here only to the extent that we cannot understand prescriptions for adequacy until we are clear about the values, ideology and objective interests and objectives of those who are prescribing for others, and the 'discourse' in which such claims are framed.[22] This naturally includes the members of governments and their current administrators who make and implement social security policy for the poor.

Governments, national or local, have many and often competing objectives. The relief of poverty may not be among the objectives of a government's social security system; if poverty is identified as a political issue at all, it is only one amongst many problems and may have little electoral importance. In reality, the making and implementation of policy are affected by a wide variety of considerations in varying political, economic and social contexts. These have been examined in Chapter 3, but it is worth remembering that for most governments managing the economy in the widest sense has generally had more political salience than have the claims of the poor.

Not only do the many competing demands on government resources at both national and local levels have to be brought forcibly together in a single budget, but an appropriate rhetoric has to be marshalled to rationalise the choices made by politicians and administrators. Even when politicians talk about justice and equity in the social security system, they may not mean combating poverty. Justice may mean social insurance provisions which give benefits related to the various levels of contributions made, or social assistance benefits according to what people are deemed to deserve. A 'just' level of compensation often depends on a person's previous position, however rich. Equity may require similar treatment for similar conditions, but it may mean different causes justify differential treatment. Neither justice nor equity may give someone an adequate social security income if they have not contributed (or sufficiently so), or if their characteristics are unacceptable, or even if they receive equitable benefits which are, however, inadequate for their needs.

When it comes to questions of what governments can afford to pay to provide adequate social security, the social security department (agency or quango) has to balance the competing demands of current or future contributors against Treasury and taxpayers, as well as current claimants. This gets even more complicated when the administering organisations are commercial firms acting as agents for government policy. Then the higher salaries for senior management and government officials, and the need for profits for shareholders, act as further constraints on benefits.

The absence of agreement on objectives can lead to much confusion in political argument about the adequacy of social security. Politicians may claim that the provisions of some income maintenance policy are 'adequate' for the objectives set for it. These objectives may be political or economic, or related to the administrative principles of the social security or taxation system in question. But at the same time the policy may be inadequate for the objective of combating poverty.

Is social security adequate in the UK?

A (very) brief history of social security adequacy standards would note that the UK's means-tested and contributory social security benefit scales have never been based on any independent evidence of what is minimally required to take part in social life, either in the long or the short term. Only one attempt has ever been made by a government department, in the 1960s, to assess the adequacy of assistance benefits. The finding that they were generally inadequate was kept secret, but only benefits for pensioners were increased as a result (Veit-Wilson, 1999). Scientific findings about poverty measures have not been used for social security, and all social security scales have been set on principles other than adequacy.

UK governments have no MIS. Instead, social security scales for people of working age have been justified by nothing more than the principle that the benefits must be held below the level of low wage rates – what has been known since the 1834 Poor Law Reform Act as the principle of 'less eligibility' (Veit-Wilson, 1989, p. 87). Since the lowest wages, even when supplemented by children's allowances, have themselves always been inadequate for social participation by families according to national standards as long as research has been carried out, see any UK survey or calculation from Rowntree (1901) to Kempson (1996), it is hardly surprising that the assistance benefits have also been inadequate for this objective.

From the beginning of the twentieth century up to the 1960s, the only standards in use in the UK were based on Seebohm Rowntree's pioneering attempts to devise prescriptive poverty measures. These were either his asocial 'primary poverty' minimum subsistence measure which he had designed to be inadequate to show disbelievers that the poor lacked enough money, not will-power, to escape poverty (Rowntree, 1901; and see Veit-Wilson, 1986), or his 'Human Needs of Labour' prescription for minimum wage rates (Rowntree 1918 and 1937).

Others then used them to count the poor, although because they were too low for adequacy they underestimated the numbers. The Beveridge Committee in 1942, making recommendations for social security benefit levels, adopted a variant of the 1901 primary poverty measure and claimed that it was enough 'for subsistence in all normal cases' (Beveridge, 1942, p. 122). Many then seemed to have overlooked the reference to subsistence and thought this meant social adequacy (Veit-Wilson, 1992; 1994).

However, in the absence of allowances to vary the family benefit according to the number of dependent children, minimum adequacy levels for social security always foundered on the less-eligibility principle. The first UK attempt to set national means-tested assistance scales, for the unemployed in 1934, was explicitly based on nothing more defensible than this principle because:

> there was no scientific standard for the calculation of all the needs to be covered by the Board; the matter was one of social convention and expediency. The Office had therefore proceeded on the principle of less eligibility; they had tried to produce a scale under which, for the ordinary family of man, wife and 3 children who had no resources, the allowance would be below net wages without having to call into operation the wage stop clause.
> (Unemployment Assistance Board Minutes 13.9.34, quoted in Veit-Wilson, 1992, p. 288)

As far as reference to setting adequacy standards was concerned, nothing changed between this date and the Department of Health and Social Security's assertion in 1979:

> The real policy decisions have been to move Supplementary Benefit rates in line with National Insurance Rates. These in turn have moved in line with movements in prices or earnings – but on quite different assumptions about the relationship between benefits and earnings than might apply for coherently developed policy on income levels necessary to combat poverty.
> (DHSS, 1979, p. 89; see also Bradshaw and Lynes, 1995)

A former Permanent Secretary of DHSS reported that until he retired in 1987 there continued to be, as in 1934, no scientific (as opposed to political) basis for the level of the social security benefit scales (Veit-Wilson, 1999, p. 118).

The situation in the 1990s is, then, that the UK social security benefit levels are not now and never have been based on any conception of adequacy in the terms with which this chapter is concerned. But that does not necessarily mean that they were or are inadequate. To find out if they are adequate, we must seek evidence from independent surveys which use defensible standards of adequacy to compare with the benefit levels, or with the levels of living actually experienced by people dependent on the social security benefits. Information about the adequacy of social security in terms of *participatory* standards comes from surveys which discover the income levels at which what society defines as minimum participatory levels of living are actually pursued, and which then compare them with the level of cash benefits.

Empirical surveys

Two national UK surveys of poverty, that of Townsend and his colleagues in 1969 (Townsend, 1979), and Mack and Lansley's in 1983 (1985), both calculated the adequacy of social assistance in terms of the poverty thresholds they discovered. Both found that the prevailing social assistance benefit levels were only about two-thirds to three-quarters of what would be required for minimal participation. In spite of much methodological qualification and argument, no contrary evidence of adequacy has been produced.

Townsend and his colleagues also carried out a study in 1985–86 in London which compared the social assistance benefit levels with the minimum income levels discovered by statistical analysis to correlate with avoiding multiple deprivations and with the levels which respondents reported as the minimum required to avoid poverty (using attitudinal measures of income adequacy). They found a high degree of agreement between the self-assessed minimum incomes and the findings of their sophisticated statistical techniques.[23] The social assistance rates were found to be only half to two-thirds of the income required for minimal adequacy (Townsend, 1993, pp. 61–62).

Normative studies

The University of York Family Budget Unit carried out studies of 'modest but adequate' and 'low cost' budgets for a range of household types in the early 1990s. The budgets were based on empirical studies of actual consumption patterns in order to capture social convention, but adjusted in order to meet prescribed standards (for instance, of nutrition or housing space). The 'modest but adequate' budget was not intended to represent a participatory minimum but in fact its components had been compared closely with the empirically derived Mack and Lansley standard of what a majority of the population defined as necessities. The 'low cost' budget was adjusted downwards by choosing fewer and lower priced goods and services and extending their lives. This resulted in an arguably poor level of living by current UK standards. Nevertheless, comparison of the 'low cost' budgets with the social assistance benefit levels for different household types showed that social assistance was adequate only for single pensioners in local authority rented housing. The benefits for all other household types were only around three-quarters of this minimally adequate standard (Yu in Bradshaw, 1993, p. 212).

Other approaches

There is a large body of accumulated evidence over many years, too extensive to cite in detail here, that most people living on the low social security and assistance benefits or on low earnings in the UK are not able to enjoy minimally adequate social participation according to conventional standards. While this body of evidence illustrates inadequacy, it does not explain where adequacy would lie. Nor do the studies of the changing relationships between the incomes of the population as a whole and those of the poorest, even though they may suggest where problems of inadequate resources might be found.

Official UK approaches to adequacy questions

Since the inception of a national social assistance scheme in the UK, poverty has persisted because of official endorsement of less eligibility in income maintenance combined with the failure to ensure that the lowest earnings were adequate, in themselves or through supplementation. Issues of adequacy in terms of participation were being recognised privately within the governmental system from the 1960s but no government considered them sufficiently salient to implement adequacy policies.

In one of its final reports, the official Supplementary Benefits Commission (SBC) expressed the view that 'To keep out of poverty, [assistance claimants] must have an income which enables them to participate in the life of the community', and gave examples of what this meant in terms of both level and tone, including full social life and the avoidance of shame and the ability 'to live in a way which ensures ... that public officials ... treat them with the courtesy due to every member of the public' (SBC, 1979, p. 2). But the SBC was abolished by the incoming Conservative government of 1979.

Since then, government ministers and officials have claimed that no independent measure of minimal adequacy is possible since all such expressions reflect nothing more than individual subjective opinion about points on an elastic continuum of tolerable inequalities (DHSS, 1985; DSS, 1989; Moore, 1989). Their conclusion that poverty no longer exists in the UK thus implies that all forms of income maintenance must be adequate, though the criteria for this judgement have not been revealed.

Conclusion

The answer to setting adequate levels is clearly complicated. The first essential is to know what adequacy means in a specific society in terms of the four questions above. That is a matter for scientific research. Much of this is still unmapped territory, even in those countries in which there has been some research on their poverty lines. Inadequate social security is not inevitable, and governments can and do pay adequate benefits in some other countries. Dutch experience in the 1970s showed that income maintenance levels could be set above the prevailing attitudinal poverty line (Goedhart *et al.*, 1977). Some Nordic countries have a statutory obligation to pay social assistance benefits which would be considered reasonable for maintaining the level of living of the population as a whole. Since the beginning of the 1980s, there have been official studies of minimum income standards in at least six countries (Australia, Belgium, Germany, New Zealand, Sweden, USA). All showed that the level and tone of benefits are consequences of political decisions which themselves arise from the interaction of government ideology with the politically salient constraints of the moment.

In modern society the state has the power to abolish poverty, even if governments do not want to accept the responsibility or use power for that purpose. Governments may not know or care where the boundaries of poverty are. If they do, they may not use them to set their own standards of minimal adequacy for income maintenance. And even if they have such standards they may not use them to determine the cash levels of any or all parts of the income maintenance system – minimum wages, tax thresholds or social security benefits. Prevailing values about the urgency of combating the poverty of all inhabitants of a country may be in conflict; the degree of social stratification may inhibit sufficient concern about the level of living and exclusion of those on the lowest incomes.

If one believes that identifying the problem of poverty inherently implies an imperative to combat it, the first requisite is clarity about the issues involved. This chapter has tried to address some of them. Dynamic standards of adequacy for the various social security and other provisions are indispensable, first as aspirations and later for monitoring continuing effectiveness in achievement. Because of the UK's experience of government neglect of these issues over decades, it is easy to become despondent about the potential for action. But the examples from other countries show that a search for adequacy standards and plans for implementing them need not be seen as naïvely utopian.

Notes

1 Note that this is a wider category than that of citizens. If all human beings matter, caring for them cannot be confined only to those who have national citizenship or residence permits, however defined.

2 Richard Titmuss's phrase.

3 Though by no means all; many people continue to find personal purchasing power inappropriate as a means of access to meaningful human relationships, and its role in meeting a person's needs for health care or education is politically contentious in the UK.

4 This fundamental point is often forgotten by those who try to specify human needs starting with material resources such as food or shelter, as if these were the most basic in defining and maintaining humanity.

5 This point is often misunderstood by those who think that 'relativity' means purely subjective opinions or distributive percentages. In fact, their assertions about 'absolute' needs are often nothing more than expressions of their own subjective views. A scientific observer might discover that in a given social context a certain resource is an 'absolute' necessity to achieve the desired social objective, but over time and in other contexts the form of that specified resource might change, relatively.

6 Note that what is socially needed is not the abstraction 'food' but the right kind of conventionally eaten food served in the right way. For detailed scholarly discussions of issues surrounding the question of human needs, see for instance Doyal and Gough (1991), or Ware and Goodin (1990).

7 Consider for example the arguments about whether anything more than temporary provision is justified for migrants, because it might encourage settlement instead of return.

8 Such as the fixed and running costs of the provision including depreciation, plus interest on capital employed and perhaps a profit element (more rarely a contribution to the wider environmental and other external costs). The prior costs of having trained staff available for hire are rarely included but should not be forgotten.

9 The question of whether saving for 'luxuries' such as holidays are to be included is a different one, considered under the heading of 'adequacy for whom?'.

10 Which was called Supplementary Benefit between the end of the National Assistance scheme in 1966 and the introduction of Income Support in 1988.

11 Germany uses studies of the actual expenditure patterns of low-earning households; Sweden uses constructed budgets for the costs of minimally adequate levels of living.

12 Finland, Norway and Sweden were studied. The requirement is written into law in the latter two countries.

13 A Dutch survey in the mid-1970s found the statutory minimum wage was higher than the national attitudinal poverty line (Goedhart *et al.*, 1977). And why should it not always be so?

14 Note also that the ideologists of both left and right who do not share the *a priori* belief in the value of individual humans, are prepared to sacrifice some of them in the interests of what they see as a greater good, whatever name they may give it. The assertions that minimum wages or Income Support benefits must be kept below the minimally adequate level 'in the interests of the country or the economy' are examples of such vicarious sacrifice. It is pointless to ask in response whose country it is or in whose interest the economy is managed by the government; the answer clearly excludes the poor.

15 A banal truism at the level of democratic electoral politics, but curiously opposed by some ostensible 'democrats' when it comes to setting standards of adequacy.

16 Just what the UK government wants long-term dependants on Income Support to do.

17 The Parker Morris Report (CHAC, 1961). A later Conservative government abandoned these standards on the grounds that they could no longer be afforded. There was no empirical evidence that social decency standards had fallen, but the government abandoned egalitarian standards and adopted stratified approaches in which public housing standards had to be 'less eligible' than private sector house-building which did not meet Parker Morris standards.

18 This was widely held to have helped to break down previous public acquiescence in the bureaucratic and personally inconsiderate way in which public services and nationalised industries were administered. Whether or not the levels of benefits were adequate, their tone certainly was not.

19 Political credibility − or perhaps expediency − can be strongly antagonistic to scientific validity. The widespread belief (at least among right-wing politicians in the UK) in the existence of an 'underclass' or a 'dependency culture' among the long-term unemployed and single mothers continues to be completely unsupported by all research, which instead shows the 'normality' of the values of the people who are suffering greatly (to the extent of serious ill health) from the lack of adequate social security in the UK. The latest study to show this, from the respected Policy Studies Institute, is Kempson *et al.* (1994). See also Cohen *et al.* (1992) and Walker (1993).

20 A notable example in discussion of the adequacy of social security is Ray's paper with that title (1993). He lists seven criteria, three of which are value statements about the level and tone of social security, but he then conflates these with four which are about government strategies to control the behaviour of the poor.

21 'Power over resources through time' and ensuring that the costs of diswelfares 'are not allowed to lie where they fall' were both expressions of the

doyen of British social policy analysts, Richard Titmuss (1907–73). His values were humanistic, egalitarian and solidaristic.

22 Discourse in this technical sense refers to the package of paradigmatic ideas and the vocabulary with which they are expressed. Discourses can be in conflict as more or less plausible to competing groups; one may be dominant to the effective exclusion of others in a country's political arguments, or be widely accepted as the prevailing wisdom without totally silencing another. Examples are the historicist/centralist discourse used in former communist countries, or the individualist/economistic discourse favoured by the 'New Right' and dominant in the UK and USA in the 1980s.

23 Except for couples under 60 without dependent children.

References

Beveridge, W.H. (1942) *Social Insurance and Allied Services*, Cmd 6404, London; HMSO.

Bradshaw, J. (ed.) (1993) *Budget Standards for the United Kingdom*, Aldershot: Avebury.

Bradshaw, J. and Lynes, T. (1995) *Benefit Uprating Policy and Living Standards*, York: Social Policy Research Unit.

Brown, M. and Madge, N. (1982) *Despite the Welfare State: A Report on the ESRC/DHSS Programme of Research into Transmitted Deprivation*, London: Heinemann.

CHAC (1961) *Homes for Today and Tomorrow*, Parker Morris, chairman, London: HMSO.

Cohen, R., Coxall, J., Craig, G. and Sadiq-Sangster, A. (1992) *Hardship Britain: Being Poor in the 1990s*, London: Child Poverty Action Group

DHSS (1979) *Social Security Research: The Definition and Measurement of Poverty*, London: HMSO.

—— (1985) *Reform of Social Security: Programme for Change*, Cmnd 9518, London: HMSO.

Doyal, L. and Gough, I. (1991) *A Theory of Human Need*, London: Macmillan.

DSS (1989) 'Benefit levels and a minimum income,' in House of Commons Social Services Committee, *Minimum Income: Memoranda laid before the Committee*, HoC Paper 579, London: HMSO.

Dubnoff, S. (1985) 'How much income is enough? Measuring public judgements,' *Public Opinion Quarterly* 49(3): 285–299.

EC (1992) 'Council Recommendation of 24 June 1992 on common criteria concerning sufficient resources and social assistance in social protection systems (92/441/EEC),' *Official Journal of the European Communities*, L(245 26 August): 46–48.

Falkingham, J. and Hills, J. (eds) (1995) *The Dynamic of Welfare: The Welfare State and the Life Cycle*, London: Prentice-Hall.

Fox, A. (1979) 'A note on industrial relations pluralism', *Sociology* 13(1): 106–109.

Goedhart, T., Halberstadt, V., Kapteyn, A. and van Praag, B. (1977) 'The poverty line: concept and measurement', *Journal of Human Resources* 12(4): 503–520.

Gordon, D. and Pantazis, C. (1997) 'Measuring poverty: Breadline Britain in the 1990's', in D. Gordon and C. Pantazis (eds) *Breadline Britain in the 1990s*, Aldershot: Ashgate, Chapter 1.

Guibentif, P. and Bouget, D. (1997) *Minimum Income Policies in the European Union*, Lisbon: União das Mutualidades Portuguesas.

Hills, J. (1995) *Joseph Rowntree Foundation Inquiry into Income and Wealth, Volume 2: A Summary of the Evidence*, York: Joseph Rowntree Foundation.

Huby, M. and Dix, G. (1992) *Evaluating the Social Fund*, London: HMSO.

Kempson, E. (1996) *Life on a Low Income*, York: York Publishing Services for the Joseph Rowntree Foundation.

Kempson, E., Bryson, A. and Rowlingson, K. (1994) *Hard Times? How Poor Families Make Ends Meet*, London: Policy Studies Institute.

Mack, J. and Lansley, S. (1985) *Poor Britain*, London: Allen and Unwin.

Maslow, A.H. (1943) 'A theory of human motivation', *Psychological Review* 50: 370–396.

Moore, J. (1989) 'The end of the line for poverty,' speech delivered by the Rt Hon John Moore MP, Secretary of State for Social Security, to the Greater London Area CPC, 11 May 1989.

Ray, J-C. (1993) 'An introductory note on measuring the adequacy of social security', in J. Berghman and B. Cantillon (eds) *The European Face of Social Security*, Aldershot: Avebury, Chapter 6.

Rowntree, B.S. (1901) *Poverty: A Study of Town Life*, London: Macmillan.

—— (1918) *The Human Needs of Labour*, London: Longmans Green.

—— (1937) *The Human Needs of Labour*, London: Longmans.

Runciman, W.G. (1972) *Relative Deprivation and Social Justice*, Harmondsworth: Penguin.

Supplementary Benefits Commission (1979) *Annual Report 1978*, Cmnd 7725, London: HMSO.

Titmuss, R. M. (1958) 'The social division of welfare: some reflections on the search for equity', in *Essays on 'the Welfare State'*, London: Allen and Unwin.

Townsend, P. (1954) 'Measuring poverty', *British Journal of Sociology* 5(2): 130–137.

—— (1962) 'The meaning of poverty', *British Journal of Sociology* 18(3): 210–227.

—— (1979) *Poverty in the United Kingdom*, Harmondsworth: Penguin.

—— (1993) *The International Analysis of Poverty*, London: Harvester Wheatsheaf.

Townsend, P. and Gordon, D. (1993) 'What is enough? The definition of a poverty line', in P. Townsend (ed.) *The International Analysis of Poverty*, London: Harvester Wheatsheaf.

Valentine, C. (1968) *Culture and Poverty*, Chicago: University of Chicago Press.

Van den Bosch, K. (1993) 'Poverty measures in comparative research', in J. Berghman and B. Cantillon (eds) *The European Face of Social Security*, Aldershot: Avebury, Chapter 1.

Veit-Wilson, J.H. (1986) 'Paradigms of poverty: a rehabilitation of B. S. Rowntree', *Journal of Social Policy* 15(1): 69–99.

—— (1989) 'The concept of minimum income and the basis of Income Support', in House of Commons Social Services Committee, *Minimum Income: Memoranda laid before the Committee*, House of Commons Paper 579, London: HMSO, pp. 74–95.

—— (1992) 'Muddle or mendacity? The Beveridge Committee and the poverty line', *Journal of Social Policy* 21(3): 269–301.

—— (1994) ' "Condemned to deprivation?" Beveridge's responsibility for the invisibility of poverty', in J. Hills, J. Ditch and H. Glennerster (eds) *Beveridge and Social Security: An International Retrospective*, Oxford: Clarendon Press, Chapter 7.

—— (1998) *Setting Adequacy Standards: How Governments Define Minimum Incomes*, Bristol: The Policy Press.

—— (1999) 'The National Assistance Board and the "rediscovery" of poverty', in H. Fawcett and R. Lowe (eds) *Welfare Policy in Britain: The Road from 1945*, London: Macmillan, Chapter 7.

Waldegrave, C. and Frater, P. (1996) 'New Zealand: a search for a poverty line', in E. Øyen, S. M. Miller and S. A. Samad (eds) *Poverty: A Global Review. Handbook on International Poverty Research*, Oslo: Scandinavian University Press, Chapter 10.

Walker, C. (1993) *Managing Poverty: The Limits of Social Assistance*, London: Routledge.

Walker, R. with Ashworth, K. (1994) *Poverty Dynamics: Issues and Examples*, Aldershot: Avebury.

Ware, A. and Goodin, R. E. (eds) (1990) *Needs and Welfare*, London: Sage.

5   British pensions policies

Evolution, outcomes and options

Eileen Evason

Introduction

This chapter examines three main questions. First, what are the options for policy-makers generally with regard to the structure and financing of provisions for persons of retirement age? Second, what tensions have shaped the evolution of pensions policy in Britain? Third, to what extent are current policies adequate to the task of meeting the needs of existing and future pensioners bearing in mind, in particular, the different life patterns of women and the radical changes occurring in the labour market? Before turning to these questions the reasons why pensions dominate debates on social security and the systems themselves are briefly considered.

The importance of pensions

Provisions for persons of retirement age are of critical and central importance in the social security systems of all industrialised countries. The centrality of this area of provision derives from a number of factors. First and foremost, there is the size of the population to be provided for and the consequent scope and cost of provision. In all industrialised countries the elderly now form a significant proportion of the population. In Britain persons of pensionable age accounted for 16.5 per cent of the population in 1991 compared with 11.4 per cent fifty years earlier (Hills, 1993, p. 31). In 1995 10.2 million persons in Britain were in receipt of state retirement pensions. The next largest group of claimants (6.9 million) was for Child Benefit (DSS, 1996). In all, in 1995–96 payments to those of pensionable age accounted for £38.8 billion – 44 per cent of total social security expenditure. The next largest item consisted of benefits for sickness and disability which totalled £22 billion (ibid.).

Second, benefits relating to retirement differ from other parts of the benefits system inasmuch as most people expect to reach retirement age and to be able to rely on the provision made for however many years they subsequently enjoy. Other groups in receipt of benefits, such as the unemployed and lone parents, may be expected and encouraged to secure the bulk of their income from earnings at some point but such assumptions have little relevance in pensions policy. Moreover, while provision for some groups constitutes a small addition to other resources, for retired persons, pensions, from whatever source, will make up the bulk of their income. On average, in Britain in 1993 only a fraction (5 per cent) of the gross income of pensioners was derived from earnings. Benefits accounted for 53 per cent and public and private sector occupational pensions for 25 per cent of average gross income (ibid.).

Pensions also stand out from other elements in income maintenance policies for a variety of other reasons. Traditionally, of all of the groups at risk of poverty, pensioners have been those most likely to be viewed as deserving of support by the general population. For governments concerned to cut or constrain costs the retired pose considerable difficulty. The unemployed may be stigmatised as work shy and the sick as malingerers but it is much more difficult to construct, and secure popular endorsement of, negative stereotypes of pensioners. However, as unemployment and job instability amongst the young increase, their circumstances may be contrasted with the security a proportion of pensioners enjoy brought by past periods of full employment and, for some, generous occupational pensions. The outlines of a strategy setting young against old are starting to emerge therefore.

A further special aspect of pensions policy relates to gender. A peculiarity of pensions policies in many countries is that they are constructed, to a large extent, for men whereas the majority of pensioners are likely to be women. In consequence, there is a sense in which policies cannot produce sensible answers because they start from the wrong questions. The key issue is typically seen as how men on average wages will fare under this or that scheme rather than how women, with very different employment patterns over life and periods of no earnings and low earnings, will be catered for (Lister, 1992 and 1994).

Finally, in the British context in particular, a further element which distinguishes pensions from other sets of benefits relates to the power and influence of non-statutory providers. The pensions industry in Britain is the major source of funds for investment. Those managing the assets of pension funds effectively control the bulk of shares in British industry and in 1991 the value of pension rights in occupational pension schemes represented one quarter of the value of all personal wealth (DSS, 1994, p. 6). The fact that the industry sits at the centre of every debate on pensions in Britain has had a significant impact on the development of policy, helps to account for the differences between provision in Britain and other European countries and has helped to turn pensions into the fault line in the broader ideological debate on the respective roles of the state and the private sector in income maintenance.

Options and choices

Structure

Before turning to the evolution of pensions policy in Britain and current debates it may be useful to try to summarise the different approaches which may be adopted, and the core questions that have to be resolved, in the construction of pensions policies generally. With regard to statutory provision there are three core options.

First, provision may consist of means-tested aid only. The obvious reasons for adopting this option are those of keeping down costs, limiting redistribution of income and avoiding long-term commitments. It should be noted that there is some room for variation within this pattern. Means tests in Britain are identified with stringency and efforts to confine assistance to all but the poorest. However, means tests may be designed instead to keep out the most affluent. In Australia the means test for the pension introduced in 1908 was steadily liberalised in subsequent decades and, although the trend was reversed in the 1980s, by 1978 the pension was approaching universal coverage with the majority (78 per cent) of persons in the eligible age group qualifying for assistance (Borowski, 1991).

The obvious disadvantage of means-testing is that to a greater or lesser extent, depending on the stringency of the means test used, it may deter people from making provision for old age. In addition, raising substantial sums from the working population without offering any benefit in return may be difficult and as living standards rise there may be less tolerance of limited provision for the retired. The options then on offer are flat rate benefits or fully earnings related benefits. Flat rate pensions may be awarded either on the basis of citizenship – the Scandinavian model – or social insurance contributions – the Beveridge model. The former has the advantages of simplicity and the provision of a floor below which the living standards of pensioners cannot fall.

Moreover, as comparative analysis (Walker, 1993; Hutton and Whiteford, 1994) demonstrates, this form of provision is particularly advantageous for women as the factors which may reduce entitlement under insurance schemes have no bearing on the pension awarded. A further potential attraction is the possibility of financing such provision out of progressive taxation. The advantages of contributory flat rate pension schemes are less clear. In the past the main strength of this strategy rested on the belief, always debatable, that contributions produced some form of contract between the individual and the state. Contributors were thought to be guaranteed benefits by virtue of their contributions. This assumed relationship helped to offset the obvious weaknesses of this model: the regressive nature of flat rate contributions and the inadequacy of benefits for those with deficient contribution records. The cuts and amendments to National Insurance benefits made by the British government during the 1980s have, however, severely undermined the general credibility of this model of provision.

Within the flat rate model the other main variation relates to adequacy. Much depends on the financial arrangements but clearly flat rate insurance benefits funded, in the main, by flat rate contributions will be limited benefits. The level of contributions will be determined by the maximum that can be imposed on those on low earnings. Universal pensions are not subject to such constraints and have, in practice, been rather more generous than British provision. Thus, in 1971 the British pension for a married couple was 26 per cent of average male earnings compared with 48 per cent in the Netherlands (Wilson, 1974, p. 349). In 1984, when the flat rate pension in Britain was starting to fall as a proportion of earnings (see below) the minimum pensions of the Nordic countries provided an income equivalent to 45 per cent of the average income of industrial workers (Knudsen, 1990).

The third option is the West European occupationally based model of earnings-related provision whereby pensions are based on past earnings and years of employment (for example, France and Germany). There is the possibility of substantial variation here with regard to the treatment of earnings, the proportion of the wage replaced and the years on which the calculation of average earnings is based. Leaving these issues aside, from a general perspective this approach may be viewed as attractive as it moves social security systems beyond the narrow focus of preventing poverty and towards the broader idea of enabling pensioners to enjoy a standard of living which in some way relates to that secured while working. Alternatively, such provision may be viewed as simply perpetuating earlier inequalities into old age. This may, in fact, be the objective. The strict proportionality of the West German scheme in its original form in 1957, which made no provision for dependent spouses and no concessions to lower paid workers, reflected a view that pensions should underwrite the value placed on people by the market. In theory, these difficulties can be overcome by the manipulation of the formula for the calculation of benefit. For example, lower paid workers may be awarded a higher proportion of previous earnings than those on average earnings and women can be credited with earnings for periods outside the labour force due to caring responsibilities. In practice, the concessions to women in particular tend to be limited.

Once a basic non-means-tested system is in place, there has been a tendency for a second layer of supplementary schemes based on past earnings and employment to develop. Within the European Union eight countries have statutory schemes with compulsory membership for some groups, while in the remaining seven supplementary provision is a matter for negotiation between employers and employees (European Commission, 1995, p. 27). Additionally, governments may encourage individuals to make further private provision.

Within this general pattern it is perhaps the UK which now provides the main exception to the rule inasmuch as there is an explicit commitment to devolving responsibility for second tier provision to the private sector and allowing the basic pension to decline. Thus, while in the rest of the European Union the private sector is still viewed as a supplement to statutory provision, UK policy implies a reversal of these roles. Indeed, in many respects the tone of recent British policy has been closer to the privatisation policies implemented in some Latin American countries which have been strongly supported by the World Bank (1994) but subject to substantial criticism from other quarters (Beattie and McGillivray, 1996; Singh, 1996).

Finance and private provision

These developments lead to consideration of two further issues in pensions policies generally: finance and the role of the private sector. With regard to finance the division is between pay-as-you-go, whereby pensions are financed from direct transfers of income between generations, and the payment of pensions from the funds accumulated through the contributions paid and the interest earned from their investment. The former tends to be identified with statutory provision and the latter with occupational and personal pensions but this distinction is not entirely satisfactory. Occupational pensions for public sector employees may, or may not, be funded. In the UK to a large extent they are not. Additionally, the French complementary schemes, which originated in the 1950s from agreements between employers and employees and thus appeared to correspond to British funded, private occupational pension schemes, operated on a pay-as-you-go basis from the start (Lynes, 1967).

Leaving aside these complications, in practice, in British debates funding has been identified with the private sector and the virtues attached to such provision relate very much to this pattern of finance. In practice, it may also be said that objective assessment of the merits of funding versus pay-as-you-go may be difficult. These issues are part and parcel of broader ideological positions which leave little room for a more pragmatic approach recognising that the appropriate strategy may vary across time depending on circumstances (Reynaud, 1995).

A central aspect of the case for funding is that this method of finance can cope more easily with demographic change. Provision has been made so an increase in the number of pensioners does not mean a rising burden on those of working age. Additionally, as the contributions are invested this may be said to be beneficial to the economy and each generation making its own provision may be seen as more virtuous than transfer arrangements whereby those of working age stake a claim to a share of the income of future workers.

There are some difficulties with all of these arguments. First, all pension arrangements represent claims on future wealth. They must be paid for out of profits or taxation (for a fuller discussion, see Downs, 1997). Second, the notion of those making private provision standing on their own two feet, rather than depending on others, is not entirely satisfactory. The cost of private pensions also falls to some extent on taxpayers via the various tax and other incentives available. The volume of such support in the UK currently stands at roughly £13 billion (DSS, 1998) and may be considered to be a particularly ill-targeted subsidy. Third, the economic argument deserves further scrutiny. As the European Commission (1995, p. 37) has noted, this form of provision may be to the detriment of the national economy if the funds for investment are channelled abroad. Alternatively, the national economy may be weakened as the pensions industry may represent a source of pressure for profits to be disbursed in the form of dividends rather than investment in new technology and training. The contrast for much of the post-war period between West Germany with a strong economy, high levels of investment and a generous pay-as-you-go pension scheme and Britain with low levels of investment, a weak economy and accumulated pension funds larger than in the rest of the European Union put together is relevant here. Finally, transfers between generations can be more positively presented as an expression of solidarity between generations to promote social cohesion with those of working age guaranteeing the position of those on whose efforts current wealth is built.

Further difficulties relate to inflation, efficiency, adequacy and predictability. In Western Europe funding was discredited by high inflation in the inter-war years. There is no guarantee that the pension obtained from funding will provide purchasing power equivalent to that forgone. Additionally, private sector funded schemes are less cost-effective than statutory pay-as-you-go schemes. Whereas administrative costs for the latter tend to be under 5 per cent of income, in the private sector charges and costs tend to absorb over 20 per cent of contributions paid in. Beyond these issues, statutory pay-as-you-go schemes provide the widest pooling of risks permitting compensation for class and gender inequalities. Such provision also has the capacity for setting precise objectives with regard to the standard of living to be afforded to pensioners. In pure, funded schemes outcomes depend on the performance of investments over very long periods of time plus the competence and honesty of advisers and those managing the funds. In addition, there is no scope for low paid workers in one scheme to be subsidised by the better paid in another or of account being taken generally of the different life patterns of women.

Finally, it should be noted that the quality and feasibility of private provision depends also on the type of provision made. In occupational pension schemes contributions may be paid by both employers and employees. The majority of such schemes in Britain award pensions based on final salary and employers may, or may not, make additional provision for post-retirement increases. The development of these schemes owes much to concern amongst employers to attract and retain key employees in past times of full employment. With high unemployment and the growth of self-employment and temporary employment, compounded by the decline of public sector schemes as a result of privatisation and competitive tendering, occupational pension schemes are likely to be of declining significance and private provision is increasingly likely to take the form of personal pensions. Here the contributions of the individual are invested and used on retirement to purchase an annuity, i.e. an annual income. Without substantial subsidy, periods of low pay and no pay will significantly depress outcomes. In 1994 the cost of provision to produce an annual income of £9,000 in the year 2020 was calculated to be £2,080 per annum for 25 years – one seventh of average net earnings at a time when the majority earned less than this (Hutton, 1995, p. 198) and few in the future will have the unbroken employment record the calculation presupposes. Not only may such provision be impractical therefore for the majority of the employed there is the issue of whether the economy could cope with the demand for dividends that such a strategy would produce.

To round off this discussion two final observations should be made. First, despite the difficulties of funding, there is a growing interest in this mechanism beyond those who would have traditionally supported this approach. Pay-as-you-go finance is subject to the hazard of growing resistance amongst those of working age to paying the contributions required in an ageing society. Moreover, pensions on this basis are vulnerable – they are more difficult to ring fence against abrupt changes in government policy. Second, however, while it is comparatively easy to move from funded to pay-as-you-go schemes, moving quickly in the reverse direction is more problematic as this entails those of working age paying for current pensions as well as making their own provision. The total cost may well exceed the projected increase in contributions which provoked the move in the first place.

The evolution of pensions in Britain

Public pensions were first introduced in Britain under the 1908 Old Age Pensions Act. The Act was preceded by a protracted debate the end result of which was a pension of five shillings a week with a test of morals as well as means attached. The cost of the pension was further curtailed by making it payable only to persons aged 70 and over. Despite its meagreness the pension was a popular measure detached as it was from the stigma of the Poor Law. It should be noted that the objective of building widows pensions into the 1911 Insurance Act was not achieved as a result of the opposition of the insurance industry which feared such provision might affect sales of policies providing lump sums on death (Gilbert, 1966).

Provision for widows did not develop until 1925 when it formed part of the broader Widows, Orphans and Old Age Pensions Act. This provided pensions of 10 shillings a week without a test of means for persons insured under the health insurance part of the 1911 Act. The same amount was payable to the widows of insured persons. The Act served to contain pressure to extend the 1908 Act and limit redistribution of income between the classes. Contributions from the young working class would support the elderly working class. In 1940 the Old Age and Widows Pensions Act amended the age at which pensions were payable to women insured in their own right and to the wives of insured males. In addition, the Unemployment Assistance Board was renamed the Assistance Board and took over responsibility from local public assistance committees for providing means-tested help for old age pensioners and widows over the age of 60. The degree of hidden poverty among the elderly was evident from the fact that, while the Board took over 250,000 cases from the public assistance committees, 'the number of pensioners who applied for and obtained a supplementary pension was considerably greater' (Beveridge, 1942, p. 213).

The result of all of this was three sets of provision, and two different means tests, which provided neither universal coverage nor adequate benefits. The solution proposed by Beveridge was flat rate, contributory pensions adequate for subsistence with a 20-year transition period. In other words the full pension would not be payable before 1965. The flat rate, subsistence approach left room for, and was in recognition of, 'the place and importance of voluntary insurance' (ibid., p. 121) and, as Glennerster (1995, p. 37) notes, Beveridge would probably never have got his proposals past the insurance lobby had he not made this clear. The Labour government decided to pay pensions at the full rate from the start but by then the full rate was barely adequate for subsistence before housing costs and a continuing and growing role for national assistance was thus guaranteed.

The post-war debate

The constant chopping and changing which have characterised British pensions policies in the post-war period derives from the continuing differences between the agendas and priorities of the two main parties. These emerged clearly in the 1950s. The Labour party focused on the inadequacy of the basic state pension and the emergence of two classes of pensioners – those in receipt of state and occupational pensions and those dependent on national assistance to top up their basic pension. There was also a growing interest in the innovative approaches to pensions provision emerging in countries such as West Germany and France. The target replacement rate of the West German scheme was 60 per cent of previous earnings and in France complementary schemes were building on the regime general which on its own had a replacement rate target of 40 per cent of earnings for those retiring at 65. British provision was beginning to seem ungenerous and outdated. By 1959 the Labour party was committed to immediate increases in flat rate benefits and their annual indexation plus the introduction of a national superannuation scheme whereby the basic pension would be augmented with an earnings-related addition. In combination, the two would provide a pension of 50 per cent of previous earnings for the employee on average wages. In line with developments in other countries, previous earnings would be dynamised, that is given their current value in the labour market, and the pension would be inflation proofed.

The Conservative government had rather different concerns which focused on limiting the nature of the basic pension, containing costs generally as the number of persons entitled to draw the basic pension increased, curtailing the contribution to the National Insurance fund from general taxation and leaving maximum scope for the development of occupational pensions. In 1953 the government appointed the Phillips Committee to review the economic and financial problems involved in providing for old age. The report of 1954 expressed approval for the growth of occupational pensions and emphasised the importance of pension funds in assisting with the shortage of capital in the post-war years. Moreover, the report helpfully concluded that the provision of a state pension for all which would be adequate for persons with no other means 'would be an extravagant use of national resources' (Phillips, 1954, p. 81). Government accepted this view at the end of 1954 and a central objective of the Beveridge Report was abandoned.

The clue to resolving the other concerns noted above was actually providing by the new thinking within the Labour party to which, with a general election imminent, the Conservative government had to respond anyway. Earnings-related pensions implied earnings-related contributions which could be used to defray the cost of flat rate benefits. The result was the graduated pension scheme introduced under the 1959 National Insurance Act. This levied additional earnings-related contributions on employees within a very narrow earnings band around the average manual worker's wage. The regressive nature of the scheme was compounded by the provisions allowing those in occupational pensions schemes to be contracted out. The extra finance would thus be raised from those who were more likely to be in low paid work. The earnings-related contributions would not, however, secure earnings-related benefits. Instead, each block of £7.50 in earnings-related contributions by male employees (£9 in the case of women), matched pound for pound by employers, would constitute a unit and the addition to the basic pension for each unit in 1994 was 7.48 pence. Finally, the very modest nature of the scheme rendered the requirement that employees could only be contracted out of the state scheme where equivalent benefits were provided of negligible significance and this left the way clear for the development of occupational pension schemes.

The pensions White Paper chase

The Labour party was in government between 1964 and 1970. Rather than proceeding immediately with the proposals already worked out for national superannuation, the government substantially increased the basic pension in 1965, with an increase in flat rate contributions, and revamped national assistance in 1966. The White Paper (DHSS, 1969) on superannuation, the Crossman plan, was published three years later. The White Paper (ibid., p. 8) stressed the high levels of dependence on means-tested benefits and the prevalence of low incomes generally amongst those of retirement age. One and a half million pensioners were in receipt of national assistance in 1965 and a further 850,000 were entitled to, but not claiming, this benefit. Moreover, if national assistance rates had been £2 higher, in that year three-quarters of pensioners would have come within the scope of the scheme.

Crossman's plan rejected reliance on occupational pensions schemes to resolve these problems pointing to the uneven coverage of this sector – only 25 per cent of employed women were in such schemes – and the limited benefits provided – 50 per cent of pensions paid in 1967 were for under £3 (ibid., p. 34). In brief, Crossman's plan was for fully earn-ings-related contributions, to be paid on wages up to a ceiling of one and a half times national average earnings, to produce an earnings-related pension weighted towards those on below average earnings. There was much emphasis in the White Paper on leaving room for occupational pension schemes but the standard they would have to meet for contracting out purposes would clearly be raised significantly.

When the Labour party lost the election in 1970, the Crossman plan fell with it. The new Conservative government was concerned to get an alternative to the Crossman scheme on to the statute book and quickly brought forward its own White Paper on pensions (DHSS, 1971). This reverted to the familiar themes of placing the basic pension on a 'sound financial basis' and 'the remarkable growth … in the provision of occu-pational pension' (ibid., paras 3 and 4). In a very decisive change of direction, the Keith Joseph plan sought to establish a clear division of labour between statutory and occupational provision. The state would be responsible for the basic pension and the provision of earnings-related pensions was to be left to occupational schemes. The only part of the Crossman scheme to survive was the notion of fully earnings related contributions which would be used to fund the flat rate pension. For those not in occupational pensions schemes, as a provision of last resort, government proposed to set up the state reserve scheme – a very basic savings scheme.

The Keith Joseph model was grounded in a determination to promote occupational pensions on the assumption that the benefits they brought to some could be extended to all. In fact, by this stage occupational pension schemes were reaching the limits of their effectiveness. In 1967 coverage peaked at 53 per cent of the labour force (it is now under 47 per cent) and the importance of such schemes in contributing to rising incomes amongst pensioners has been a consequence of the characteristics of those covered, high earners in permanent employment, rather than the private nature of these schemes (Johnson and Falkingham, 1994).

The Keith Joseph scheme did reach the statute book in 1973 but the new Labour government in 1974 repealed the legislation and brought forward its own proposals. The Castle scheme (DHSS, 1974) was less complex than Crossman's, contained something for existing as well as future pensioners and paid particular attention to the position of women. In broad outline, the new structure contained in the 1975 Pensions Act was as follows. The basic pension would continue but would be increased annually in line with prices or wages, whichever were higher. Thus the pension would move up in line with real increases in living standards amongst the working population if such occurred. As was noted above, a strong base benefits the lower paid and women. The basic pension would be supplemented by an earnings-related addition (SERPS) consisting of 25 per cent of average earnings between the base pension and an earnings ceiling with the more limited commitment that this would be inflation proofed. Past earnings would be dynamised and the average wage calculated by reference to the best twenty years across working life. Basing the additional pension on the best twenty years would reduce the effects of periods of low earnings and no earnings thus giving further recognition to the needs of women and the lower paid. With regard to women specifically, widows would fully inherit the entitlement of their husbands and, while a full basic pension would be conditional on contributions being paid or credited for the requisite years (roughly 90 per cent of working life), the requisite years would be reduced by those spent outside the labour force caring for children or others. Finally, the Castle scheme provided for employees to be contracted out of the state earnings related scheme but only if, as a minimum, contributors were guaranteed equivalent benefits. In recognition of the difficulties of occupational pensions schemes with regard to, for example, post-retirement inflation proofing, mechanisms would be introduced whereby the state would underwrite occupational provision. As Shragge notes (1984, p. 146), at a time of very high inflation this provision was of critical importance to the pensions industry. The whole scheme would come in to operation after a twenty-year transitional period commencing in 1978.

With hindsight, the Castle scheme may be criticised on a number of grounds, for example, the lowness of the earnings replacement rate for those on below average earnings and the scale and cost of the concessions to the pensions industry. Nevertheless, taken as a whole the scheme was certainly comparable with the most developed schemes in Europe and was 'the most advanced in the world in terms of equal rights for women and carers' (Glennerster, 1995, p. 114). The Bill went through Parliament with all party support and was endorsed by representatives of the pensions industry. It appeared that a consensus had finally been reached.

Pensions post-1979

The consensus did not last long. The Conservative government elected in 1979 began almost at once to dismantle the structure established by the 1975 Pensions Act. In 1980 the formula for uprating long-term benefits was amended. From 1982 the basic pension would rise in line with prices only. The implications of this were twofold. First, the basic pension would fall steadily behind earnings. In 1981 the pension was 23 per cent of average male earnings. By 1993 it was down to 15 per cent and it is projected this figure will be down to 10 per cent by 2010, at which point its abolition altogether will be possible. Second, the amendment of the uprating formula made the amendment of SERPS inevitable as part of the savings on the base would otherwise be offset by increased additional pension entitlement. The 25 per cent would be based on a larger chunk of earnings.

In 1983 government announced that an Inquiry, to be chaired by then Secretary of State, Norman Fowler, would be set up to consider the future development, adequacy and cost of pensions. As its first task the Inquiry undertook a study of personal pensions. The sudden emergence of personal pensions, and the way this option moved so quickly up the agenda in the 1980s to become the preferred model of provision, require some explanation. Nesbitt's (1995) analysis of this period, and subsequent developments, indicate that three elements were crucial. First, there was the sheer energy with which personal pensions were sold by members of radical right wing think tanks. Second, whereas occupational pensions smack of corporatism and the job for life, personal pensions, with individuals being responsible for and in control of their own provision, were much more in tune with the new individualistic culture of people's capitalism. Third, the drive towards a flexible labour market requires flexible pensions which can cope with frequent job changes. This is a difficulty for occupational pensions and if the obvious option – a state scheme – is not on the agenda, personal pensions are all that remain.

The Inquiry produced neither policy recommendations nor a consensus but it was followed by the proposal, in the broader 1985 Green Paper (DHSS, 1985a) on the restructuring of social security, to abolish SERPS altogether. For SERPS would be substituted compulsory membership of an occupational or personal pension. The proposal was defeated by the Treasury, concerned with the loss of revenue this would entail, and the pensions industry which did not wish to take responsibility for large numbers of low paid workers. The subsequent White Paper (DHSS, 1985b) proposed to retain SERPS but in a much modified form. The replacement ratio would be cut from 25 per cent to 20 per cent and calculated from earnings across the whole of working life. The average earnings figure would be depressed by periods of low earnings and no earnings and, taken together, these two changes would cut average SERPS entitlement by half. In addition, widows would inherit only half of their husband's entitlement. Most significantly, the White Paper proposed financial incentives for persons leaving SERPS to take out an approved personal pension and for members of newly contracted out occupational pensions. The standards to be met in such cases represented a distinct lowering of the quality threshold in pensions. The test related to guaranteed minimum levels of contributions – inputs rather than outcomes.

These proposals were put in place in 1986 and the changes in SERPS began to take effect in 1988. The determination of government to present SERPS as a less desirable option generally was evident in the advertising campaign launched at the time at a cost of £1 million to extol the virtues of personal pensions.

Problems and responses in the 1990s

Some of the flaws in this strategy emerged over the following five years. First, the Committee of Public Accounts (1991, para. 20) concluded that the cost of the inducements to membership of approved personal pensions was likely to be £9.3 billion while the savings to the National Insurance Fund would be £3.4 billion, making the net cost of a policy presented as reducing public expenditure £5.9 billion. Second, at the end of 1991 confidence in occupational pensions was undermined by the Maxwell scandal. Following the death of the publisher, it was discovered that £450 million had been illegally removed from the pensions funds of his companies. In an attempt to restore the image of this form of provision, the government appointed the Goode Committee to make recommendations to give greater security to the members of company pensions schemes. The Committee reported in 1993 and a White Paper (DSS, 1994) and the 1995 Pensions Act followed. Within the context of replying to the Goode report, however, the government appeared to be pursuing its broader strategy with regard to pensions.

Three points can be noted. First, the provisions put in place were a weakened version of the Goode report and will not necessarily prevent another Maxwell scandal nor significantly alter the current imbalance of power between employers and members of occupational pension schemes (Ward, 1996). Moreover, it would appear that the inadequacy of one aspect of the new arrangements has already been demonstrated. The compensation scheme will only be triggered where theft or fraud is proved and, given the acquittal of the Maxwell brothers, this provision would have been of no assistance to the Maxwell pensioners. Second, by 1994, government was concerned over the implications of rulings by the European Court of Justice requiring equal treatment of women by occupational pension schemes. The White Paper made it clear (DSS, 1994, para. 2.1) that the quid pro quo of compliance was further weakening of the standards contracted out schemes would be required to meet. From 1997 the requirement that non-money purchase occupational pension schemes provide a guaranteed minimum pension would be abolished and replaced by a general test of quality. In essence, none of the three private sector elements would have to provide assured outcomes. This will further defray the cost to the state of the underwriting provisions introduced initially under the Castle scheme and finally break the link with SERPS. The private sector is being floated off and the way was opened to further amend or abolish SERPS altogether. In a further cost saving measure in 1994 the government announced the state pension age would be raised to 65 for women. This change will affect women born after 1950.

Third, the White Paper contained proposals to give further encouragement to contracted out occupational money purchase schemes and approved personal pensions through the introduction of age-related national insurance rebates. Older workers would get greater assistance in leaving SERPS.

The continued determination to promote personal pensions is perhaps surprising as by this stage a further scandal – the mis-selling of personal pensions – had emerged. By 1994 six million people had taken out approved personal pensions. Of these, about two million had left

SERPS but would have been better advised to remain with the state scheme and half a million had left occupational pension schemes for inferior personal pensions (Hutton, 1995). The industry was exposed as driven by commission rather the best interests of customers. Two responses followed. First, the Securities and Investments Board – now the Financial Services Authority – introduced new rules requiring insurance salesmen to, for example, disclose the commission on policies sold. They are not required, however, to disclose whether this is more or less than for other policies. The need for persons to remember to ask if there is a cheaper product and shop around may be considered to be a less than satisfactory way of providing for future pensioners. Second, procedures were put in place to try to identify and compensate those affected by the scandal. The process has been slow and when and whether this whole episode will be resolved is unclear.

The case for change

The pace of change over the past decade in pensions policy has been remarkable. It is appropriate therefore to stand back to review the grounds on which such rapid and radical developments have occurred.

Taking all of the White Papers published in this period (DHSS, 1985a, 1985b; DSS, 1993a, 1993b, 1995) together, the case for this total strategy rested on a cluster of minor and more substantive arguments. In the minor category may be placed arguments relating to the needs of existing pensioners and choice. The 1985 Green Paper (DHSS, 1985a, Chapter 7) argued that it was inappropriate for those currently employed to promise themselves more generous pensions via SERPS which did nothing for existing pensioners. This perspective might have had more force if the incomes of existing pensioners had not been depressed by the amendment to the uprating formula in 1980 and the cuts in housing benefit in 1988. With regard to choice, while emphasis has been placed (DSS, 1994, p. 22) on the desirability of enabling persons to choose the pension that is best for them, under these policies choice is constrained by means and what the market offers. Given a completely free choice the self-employed person on a low income might prefer membership – which has never been open to this group – of SERPS.

More substantially, emphasis has been on projected increases in costs as the numbers of pensioners rises to 13.2 million in 2035 with a sharp fall in the ratio of pensioners to persons of working age (DHSS, 1985a, p. 15). There has been the constant assumption that social security expenditure generally (DSS, 1993a) is in danger of moving beyond what the nation can afford and it has been further argued that British policy is in line with broader trends whereby many other countries are taking steps to contain the cost of social security (DSS, 1993b).

Much of this cluster of propositions is also open to debate. First, taking radical action in the 1980s to deal with problems which might arise in the distant future may be viewed as prudence or opportunism. The Social Security Advisory Committee concluded:

> We do not feel it would be justifiable to make pension scheme changes now in anticipation of a demographic problem in fifty years time. We consider that it would be more sensible to wait until the turn of the century when not only will the likely ratio of elderly people to workers be clearer but the longer-term prospects for economic growth through into the next century will be more apparent.
>
> (1984, para. 3.9)

It should be further noted that throughout this debate there has been no indication that policy would change even if a dramatic decline in the numbers of future pensioners were suddenly forecast and the concept of dependency ratios is, perhaps, not all that helpful anyway. The crucial factors are the levels of employment, investment and productivity. A very favourable dependency ratio may still result in difficulties in paying for pensions if large numbers of those of working age are actually unemployed.

Second, following on from this, there is concern that policy has rested on worst case scenarios. The years selected represent the peak of the increase caused by the baby boom of 1960s when the dependency ratio will be at its lowest. After this the ratio will improve and the work of Hills (1993, p. 13) indicates that in the year 2040 the dependency ratio will be more favourable in the UK than in Japan, the USA and New Zealand and the most favourable in the European Union excluding the Republic of Ireland. Additionally, it has been argued (Andrews and Jacobs, 1990; Oppenheim, 1994) that the case presented has taken the most pessimistic projections of economic growth and unemployment.

Third, the notion of pensions costs rising to levels beyond the means of the nation is questionable. This was a central element in the case for amending SERPS in 1986 but it can be argued that the increase in National Insurance contributions required over time to maintain existing provision was manageable and, indeed, modest by comparison with the increases which actually occurred between 1979 and 1985 (Davies, 1993). Account should also be taken of the UK's relatively modest spending on welfare and the way in which the debate has been confined to the cost of state pensions with no attempt to make a full, value for money, assessment of the total costs of the alternatives to maintaining the basic pension and SERPS.

Finally, with regard to the international dimensions of his debate, it is true to say that other countries have been making significant adjustments to their pensions policies. In the majority of member states within the European Union a mixture of amendments can be discerned: for example, bringing the retirement age for women into line with that for men; reducing the proportion of earnings replaced and altering the years of employment on which the calculation is based (European Commission, 1995). However, while other countries have made selections from the options available, Britain has adopted virtually all of them and, in addition, moved decisively towards privatisation.

Pensioners' incomes in the 1990s and future options

The outcome for British pensioners by the early 1990s of all of the policy developments discussed in this chapter can be stated fairly briefly: 17 per cent of pensioners were in receipt of means-tested income support, 28 per cent of older people in the United Kingdom lived on or below the poverty line (Walker, 1993) and in 1988/9 33 per cent of pensioner couples and 42 per cent of single pensioners were living on incomes below 50 per cent of average incomes (DSS, 1992). Pensioners' incomes did rise faster than those of all households between 1979 and 1991–92 but this was more of a reflection of increasing inequality within the pensioner population rather than general improvement. The incomes of those with occupational pensions were higher but those without occupational pensions 'were more narrowly concentrated around the same real income level as ten years before' (Inquiry into Income and Wealth, 1995, p. 27). In essence, current patterns reflect earlier access to forms of provision that are in decline. In time, those who are more likely to have occupational pensions will replace those who are older and poorer but their place will be taken by pensioners with more variable entitlement.

With regard to the future, as things stand, British pensioners will receive nugatory basic pensions with the larger part of non means-tested income being derived from sources which reflect earlier inequalities. The work of Hills (1993) indicates that the basic pension for a person earning the male average wage in each year between 1992 and 2040 will equal 7.5 per cent of average earnings while the SERPS addition, guaranteed minimum pension in the case of contracted out employees, will amount to 13.9 per cent of average earnings. That this is all that can be relied on with certainty after so much effort is remarkable and, in any case, most people, will not have a record of continuous employment on average wages. Current policies are beginning to seem very ill suited to meeting the needs of women, those on below average earnings and the rising number of irregularly employed.

In the light of all this, a number of proposals for change had been developed by the mid-1990s. The options on offer were of varying degrees of complexity. A very basic proposal (Dilnot and Johnson, 1992) was to leave things as they were but means test the basic pension using the savings made to assist the poorest pensioners. Leaving aside the possibility that the savings will not be delivered to the poorest, this option may produce opposition from those who have paid contributions for decades and raises all of the old problems of disincentives.

A second possibility was to phase out SERPS and the subsidies to approved personal and occupational pensions and concentrate resources on improving the basic pension and moving towards provision financed from progressive taxation based on citizenship rather than insurance contributions. The pensions industry would be allotted the role of assisting those able and willing to make additional provision but would do so without subsidy. A strong universal pension would be of particular benefit to those who are likely to do badly out of current arrangements and would, at least, be comprehensible to the general public. The most obvious difficulties in the way of such a strategy are the opposition of the pensions industry, the long transitional period which would be needed by virtue of the volume of accrued rights from the existing arrangements and the difficulties of securing support for such a clearly redistributive approach.

Located somewhere between these two basic options was the concept of a pensions guarantee whereby the state ensures that the combined pension income from all sources is topped up where it falls below the prescribed levels. The advantage of this proposal is that if the prescribed levels were to be maintained in line with earnings and set above current income support levels then women, the low paid and the very elderly would gain. The losers would be those with company and personal pensions which took them above the prescribed levels. As the Commission on Social Justice (Borrie, 1994) points out, it could be argued that these groups have already received substantial state subsidy. The main difficulties with the pension guarantee are that it could easily turn into a more basic and less adequate means-tested pension and might provide an incentive for people to switch to other forms of provision outside the scope of the guarantee. Thus, compulsory membership of some form of second-tier provision would still be required.

Dealing with the disincentives of means-testing and the pensions guarantee requires more complex solutions and here, apart from leaving things as they were, a wide range of options emerged. The first possibility (Castle and Townsend, 1996) was a revitalised basic pension and the restoration of SERPS in full. It can be argued that this is the most cost-effective way of making provision which adequately responds to the needs of women and the lower paid and the implications of a flexible labour market. Much of the case for the amendments of 1986 was questionable and one of those involved has admitted that ideology, rather than demographic pressure, was the driving force behind the changes of the 1980s (Davies, 1993, p. 40). One obvious difficulty with this strategy is that it is impossible to ensure that the scheme would not be undermined once again at a later stage. Additionally, as Davies (ibid., p. 43) notes, there is the difficulty of selling a complex scheme in the face of opposition from a strong industry which devotes substantial resources to public relations.

The need to produce a scheme which people can understand and identify with, and which is not so susceptible to future manipulation, was fundamental to the proposals of Davies (1993) and Field (1993). Davies' proposal was, first, for an improved basic pension to be financed from current contributions together with the restoration of the Treasury supplement to the National Insurance Fund and the abolition of the income tax age allowance. The second tier would consist of a new version of SERPS – the National Personal Pension Scheme – with individual accounts, annual statements and nominal contributions invested in a new class of government bonds. Contracting out would be on the basis of equivalent benefits and there would be substantial reform of occupational pensions. This proposal addressed a fundamental flaw in past statutory provision: failure to involve people and provide clear information on what their contributions are used for and what they themselves can expect. It would still, however, be open to manipulation based, perhaps, on the charge, reasonable or otherwise, that it was pretending to be something that it was not.

Field's proposal appeared to deal with this problem and was based on the concept of personal pensions for all. In essence, there would be a guaranteed minimum pension which would be set at about 20 per cent above the current basic retirement pension and designed so that only the most affluent pensioners lost the larger part of their entitlement. The second tier would consist of universal personal pensions with compulsory contributions from employers and employees. The state would pay contributions for those not in paid employment. One problem with this strategy is that its adequacy hinges on the provisions for those who are normally disadvantaged by this form of provision and it is this part of the scheme which it is most difficult to guarantee. A similar difficulty arose with Johnson and Falkingham's (1994, pp. 255–270) proposals for combining all basic and secondary provision so that each individual has their own pension fund with tax financed subsidies for those on low incomes or outside the labour market altogether. More generally, these proposals for moving towards funding raise issues of time-scale and the logic and cost effectiveness of trying to provide for existing and future pensioners at the same time when the main objective, securing pensions from future interference, is probably unattainable.

Conclusion – another fresh start

At the time of going to press it would appear that the policy adopted by the Labour government consists of a curious amalgam of some of the options outlined above. The Green Paper *A New Contract for Welfare: Partnership in Pensions* (DSS, 1998) proposes a strategy with four main tiers. First, there is to be a means-tested minimum income guarantee for pensioners which, it is intended, will be increased in line with wages rather than prices. Second, the basic state pension will continue but with no alteration to the up-rating formula. Third, the objective in the long run is to convert SERPS into a flat rate Second State Pension confined to those on low earnings – under £9,000 per annum – with those caring for persons with disabilities or children under five being credited with contributions for this. Similar arrangements will operate for persons whose employment is disrupted by disability. Fourth, more generous rebates on National Insurance contributions will be available for those on modest earnings – £9,000 to £18,500 – who take out the new, funded stakeholder pensions which the government anticipates will have lower costs and be more flexible than existing personal pensions. Finally, underneath all of this is the objective of reducing state spending on pensions as a proportion of GDP from 4.4 per cent in the year 2000 to 3.4 per cent in 2050 thus reversing the current ratio whereby state provision accounts for 60 per cent of support for pensioners and the private sector 40 per cent.

There are a number of obvious potential difficulties with this strategy. First, trying to run a generous minimum income guarantee without compulsion for those on modest incomes to make additional provision beyond the basic pension may be difficult. Additionally, the strategy may give rise to confusion and annoyance amongst existing pensioners. In April 1999 the basic pension for a single person increased in line with inflation from £64.70 to £66.75. The Income Support rate – renamed the Minimum Income Guarantee – for pensioners under 75 rose more sharply from £70.45 to £75. Pensioners who thought that the much advertised increase to £75 related to the basic pension were disappointed and, when the value of the pension for which contribu-

tions have been paid falls so far behind provision for which no contributions are required, the system may be viewed as unfair.

Second, the new stakeholder pensions are a new and untried form of
provision. There is to be a 1 per cent limit on annual management fees and
providers must be willing to accept persons making contributions as low as
£10 a month with no penalties where members suspend contributions.
These conditions have been greeted with dismay amongst insurance
companies and whether other organisations will be prepared to act as
providers of these schemes on the scale anticipated by government is
unclear. Most importantly, funded personal pensions from very modest
contributions will – even if charges are minimal – produce at the very most
pensions which, for many, may hardly equal means-tested provision. We
are thus back to the problem of disincentives and it is difficult to see how
this problem can be resolved. Compelling people to make more adequate
provision via non statutory providers would be unpopular amongst those
who are hard pressed financially and would, moreover, imply some form of
state guarantee with regard to outcomes which is clearly not on the agenda.

Third, taken as a whole, the strategy fits in with the broader agenda of
government with regard to social security – the steady erosion of benefits under the National Insurance scheme with efforts being made to
protect the poorest via means-tested assistance and, to a lesser extent, by
the very narrowly circumscribed Second State Pension. Such a strategy is
highly vulnerable to change in government, or a change in government
priorities or a change in economic circumstances which requires cuts to
be found quickly. The strategy also assumes the acquiescence of those
who gain little or nothing for their National Insurance contributions.

In conclusion, whilst it is unclear at the time of writing whether
these proposals will be fully implemented, it would appear that, despite
the title of the 1998 Green Paper, we are witnessing a withdrawal of the
two key factors from the field. Employers are moving away from final
salary occupational pension schemes towards money purchase arrangements - with defined inputs rather than outputs – or no arrangements at
all. The state is seeking to reduce its role and liability. The costs and risks
are being shifted on to the individual. Overall, it would seem that the
muddle and uncertainty which have characterised British pensions
policy in this century will persist into the next.

Acknowledgements

I am grateful to Dulcie Groves, Honorary Lecturer in Social Policy,
University of Lancaster for her many helpful thoughts and comments
on the draft version of this chapter.

References

Andrews, K. and Jacobs, J. (1990) *Punishing The Poor*, London: Macmillan.

Beattie, R. and McGillivray, W. (1996) 'Rejoinder', *International Social Security Review* 49(3): 17–21.

Beveridge, W. (1942) *Social Insurance and Allied Services* Cmd 6404, London: HMSO.

Borowski, A. (1991) 'The economics and politics of retirement incomes policy in Australia', *International Social Security Review* 44(1–2): 27–41.

Borrie, G. (1994) *Social Justice Strategies For Renewal: Report of the Commission on Social Justice*, London: Vintage.

Castle, B. and Townsend, P. (1996) *We CAN Afford the Welfare State: Security in Retirement for Everyone*, London:

Committee of Public Accounts. (1991) *The Elderly: Information Requirements For Supporting The Elderly: The Implications of Personal Pensions For The National Insurance Fund*, London: HMSO.

Davies, B. (1993) *Better Pensions For All*, London: IPPR.

Department of Health and Social Security (1969) *National Superannuation and Social Insurance: Proposals For Earnings Related Social Security* Cmnd 3883, London: HMSO.

—— (1971) *Strategy For Pensions*, Cmnd 4755, London: HMSO.

—— (1974) *Better Pensions Fully Protected against Inflation*, Cmnd 5713, London; HMSO.

—— (1985a) *Reform of Social Security*, Vol. 1, Cmnd 9517, London: HMSO.

—— (1985b) *Reform of Social Security: Programme for Action*, Cmnd 9691, London: HMSO.

—— (1992) *Households Below Average Income*, London: HMSO.

Department of Social Security (1993a) *The Growth of Social Security*, London: HMSO.

—— (1993b) *Containing the Cost of Social Security: The International Context*, London: HMSO.

—— (1994) *Security, Equality, Choice: The Future for Pensions*, Vol. 1 Cm 2594.1, London: HMSO.

—— (1996) *Social Security Statistics 1996*, London: HMSO.

—— (1998a) *New Ambitions for Our Country: A New Contract for Welfare*, Cm 3805, London: HMSO.

—— (1998b) *A New Contract for Welfare: Partnerships in Pensions*, Cm 4179, London: HMSO.

Dilnot, A. and Johnson, P. (1992) 'What pensions should the state provide?', *Fiscal Studies* 13(4).

Downs, C. (1997) 'Pensions for an older population', *Benefits: A Journal of Social Security, Research, Policy and Practice* 18: 9–12.

European Commission (1995) *Europe Social Protection*, Brussels: Directorate General Employment, Industrial Relations and Social Affairs.

Field, F. (1993) *Private Pensions for All: Squaring the Circle*, Discussion Paper No. 16, London: Fabian Society.

Gilbert, Bentley B. (1966) *The Evolution of National Insurance in Great Britain*, London: Michael Joseph.

Glennerster, H. (1995) *British Social Policy Since 1945*, Oxford: Blackwell.

Goode, R. (1993) *Pensions Law Reform, Vols 1 and 2*, London: HMSO.

Hills, J. (1993) *The Future of Welfare: A Guide to the Debate*, York: Joseph Rowntree Foundation.

—— (1995) *Joseph Rowntree Foundation Inquiry into Income and Wealth*, vol. 2, York: Joseph Rowntree Foundation.

Hutton, S. and Whiteford, P. (1994) 'Gender and retirement incomes: a comparative analysis', in S. Baldwin and J. Falkingham (eds) *Social Security and Social Change*, Hemel Hempstead: Harvester Wheatsheaf.

Hutton, W. (1995) *The State We're In*, London: Jonathan Cape.

Johnson, P. and Falkingham, J. (1994) 'Is there a future for the Beveridge pension scheme?', in S. Baldwin and J. Falkingham (eds) *Social Security and Social Change*, Harvester Wheatsheaf.

Knudsen, P. (1990) 'The future of the pension system in Norway', *International Social Security Review*, 2/90: 213–227.

Lister, R. (1992) *Women's Economic Dependency and Social Security*, Manchester: Equal Opportunities Commission.

—— (1994) '"She has other duties": women, citizenship and social security', in S. Baldwin and J. Falkingham (eds) *Social Security and Social Change*, Harvester Wheatsheaf.

Lynes, T. (1967) *French Pensions,* London: Bell and Sons Ltd.

Nesbitt, S. (1995) *British Pensions Policy Making in the 1980s*, Aldershot: Avebury.

Oppenheim, C. (1994) *The Welfare State: Putting the Record Straight*, London: Child Poverty Action Group.

Phillips (1954) *Report of the Committee on the Economic and Financial Problems of the Provision Of Old Age*, Cmd 9333, London: HMSO.

Reynaud, E. (1995) 'Financing retirement pensions schemes: pay-as-you-go and funded systems in the European Union', *International Social Security Review* 48(2–4): 41–58.

Shragge, E. (1984) *Pensions Policy in Britain: A Socialist Analysis*, London: Routledge and Kegan Paul.

Singh, A. (1996) 'Pension reform, the stock market, capital formation and economic growth: a critical commentary on the World Bank's proposals', *International Social Security Review*, 49(3): 21–45.

Social Security Advisory Committee (1984) *Third Report*, London: HMSO.

Townsend, P. and Walker, A. (1996) 'The future of pensions', *Benefits: A Journal of Social Security Research, Policy and Practice*, 15.

Walker, A. (1993) 'Achieving (or not achieving) economic security in old age: The EC pension systems compared', *Benefits: A Journal of Social Security Research, Policy and Practice* 8: 4–8.

Ward, S. (1996) 'The 1995 Pensions Act', *Benefits: A Journal of Social Security Research, Policy and Practice*, 15.

Wilson, T. (ed.) (1974) *Pensions, Inflation and Growth*, London: Heinemann.

World Bank (1994) *Averting the Old Age Crisis: Policies to Protect the Old and Promote Growth*, World Bank Policy Research Report, Oxford: Oxford University Press.

6 Claiming entitlements

Take-up of benefits

Anne Corden

Introduction

Social security is effective only in so far as provision reaches those for whom it is designed. The current policy emphasis is towards allocative systems which aim to match resources to needs by selective targeting, and away from principles of universality in achieving optimal distribution. The underlying historical assumption in an allocative scheme which attempts to match resources to needs is that citizens will claim their rights, and thus responsibility for achieving a just distribution may be shared between potential beneficiaries, government and administrative agents. The balance of these responsibilities varies, however, according to the benefit and its place in the overall social security scheme. In some cases, responsibility for identifying possible eligibility and making an application lies heavily on the potential beneficiary, as with the discretionary social fund. A greater share of responsibility is usually assumed by government where a benefit has special strategic or political importance. Family credit is the prime example here. This is a rules-based benefit, with entitlement according to strict eligibility criteria, but its apparent key importance in maintaining work incentives has led government to assume responsibility for major promotional activity and investigation of ways of encouraging applications.

As might be expected in an overall system which rests on variously shared responsibilities, with assumptions about human behaviour, problems arise in achieving appropriate access. Benefits which attract relatively large proportions of applications from ineligible people are expensive to administer, and cause confusion and disappointment. Some benefits, the government believes, are apparently delivered to problematic numbers of people without entitlement. On the other hand, some benefits remain unclaimed by those who qualify to receive them, despite major administrative efforts. Non-take-up of benefits has remained high on the social security research agenda for nearly four decades, a focus of interest for both central and local government, the academic community, and those community groups and organisations that represent the interests of people who need access to financial resources.

The study of take-up of benefit is an essential component of debates about universality and selectivity in the allocation of resources, and it is worth devoting a whole chapter to this topic. There is much to learn about the way in which social security functions by looking at work that has been done in an attempt to understand differential take-up of benefits. Take-up studies bring together concerns with efficiency and effectiveness against a background of administrative complexity and claimant sensitivity. Recent work is especially important in emphasising the role of structure and systems in determining policy outcomes.

The first part of this chapter asks why take-up has traditionally received so much attention within social security policy and research. Measuring take-up is a technical issue, and the second section of the chapter explains how we estimate levels of take-up of income-related benefits. The chapter goes on to consider what has been learned about factors which influence take-up, and follows the development of ideas through a spectrum of disciplines – psychology and human behaviour, sociology, economics and social policy. People's own decision-making and behaviour are important, of course, in determining the eventual level of take-up of any particular benefit. However, recent work suggests that equal weight must be given to structural and administrative levels of influence if we are to understand what happens.

The chapter ends by looking at what has been learned from such intensive focused study over three decades, and how far policy has responded. The implications of recent research represent a powerful challenge to government policy.

The importance of take-up

The term take-up is used to describe the process of claiming entitlements to benefits. A take-up estimate is a quantified outcome measure, representing that proportion of overall entitlement actually received, or the percentage of people entitled who receive benefit. For a contributory benefit such as state retirement pension take-up is nearly 100 per cent, and as with the universal child benefit, nearly everyone with an entitlement receives what is due. Among the main income-related benefits take-up is much lower. Table 6.1 presents the most recent government estimates of income-related benefit take-up.

Table 6.1 shows the two traditional measures of take-up. The

Table 6.1 Official estimates of income-related benefit take-up, 1995–96

	Expenditure take-up	Caseload take-up
Housing benefit	93–96%	89–94%
by family type:		
lone parents	98–100%	96–100%
pensioners	89–92%	86–89%
by tenure:		
local authority tenants	94–97%	91–96%
private tenants	91–94%	86–91%
Income support	88–92%	76–82%
by family type:		
lone parents	98–100%	96–100%
pensioners	72–78%	60–66%
Family credit	83%	70%
by family type:		
lone parents	91%	80%
couples	76%	62%
Council tax benefit	76–84%	74–82%
by family type:		
lone parents	91–96%	90–96%
pensioners	68–76%	66–74%
by tenure:		
local authority tenants	90–99%	88–99%
private tenants	81–88%	79–86%
owner-occupiers	57–64%	54–61%

Source: Income Related Benefits: Estimates of Take-up in 1995/96, (DSS, 1997).

Note: Estimates are only for people living in private households, and do not include self-employed people.

expenditure-based estimate compares the amount of benefit received, in the course of a year, with the total amount that would be received if everybody took up their entitlement. The caseload-based measure compares the number of benefit recipients, averaged over the year, with the number who would be receiving if everybody took up their entitlement. Within these overall estimates, take-up measures are also available for people in different family types (DSS, 1997). Lone parents consistently show higher take-up than couples, and take-up of income support, housing benefit and council tax benefit is generally lowest among pensioners. Where take-up measures are also available by tenure type, estimates for local authority tenants are highest. Take-up is specially low among pensioners entitled to income support, at 60–66 per cent of caseload, and among owner-occupiers entitled to council tax benefit, at 54–61 per cent in 1995–96. The fact that the expenditure-based figures are consistently higher than the caseload estimates means that average awards are higher than average amounts left unclaimed, suggesting that there may be costs to claiming which outweigh the value of the benefits.

Successive governments have struggled hard to improve the take-up of these income-related benefits. Despite the huge saving to the public purse represented by these unclaimed benefits, there are several reasons for concern. The first is the link between non-take-up and poverty, which first became clear in the 1950s and early 1960s (Corden, 1983; Craig, 1991). In simple terms, people who are not claiming entitlements to minimum income provision are likely to be very poor and receipt of their entitlements might raise incomes and improve living standards. Those with unclaimed income support have financial resources below what is available as a minimum 'safety net'. The official income support take-up estimates for 1995–96 suggest, for example, that between 800,000 and 1,070,000 elderly people with entitlement were missing out, on average, on £16.10 per week, and between 10,000 and 40,000 couples with children could have had, on average, an extra £53.50 per week (DSS, 1997).

Alongside the link between poverty and non-take-up, the measures of take-up provide indicators of policy effectiveness in implementing social security policy. Benefits which are designed to target resources on the most needy people in society (DHSS, 1985) must be seen to be hitting those targets. Non-take-up is a measure of the extent to which such benefits are missing their targets, and policy is ineffective. For the government, one of the most problematic benefits in this respect has been family credit, and the similar benefit which preceded it, family income supplement (Corden and Craig, 1991). Family credit was designed to spring the unemployment trap for families with children by making parents better off in work than on out-of-work benefits. The benefit could therefore both boost low incomes and maintain work incentives. How far the benefit fulfils this role depends on how many people respond to the advantages offered in principle. A stream of research from the early 1980s has been conducted in order to understand better how people perceive and respond to this benefit, and how take-up might be increased (Callender *et al.*, 1994; Corden, 1983, 1987; Corden and Craig, 1991; Craig, 1991; Eardley and Corden, 1996; Marsh and McKay, 1993; McKay and Marsh, 1995; Noble *et al.*, 1992; Walker with Ashworth, 1994).

There are also practical reasons for wanting to know more about take-up. Before new benefits are introduced or rules of existing benefits are changed the Treasury requires accurate forecasts of numbers of people who may be eligible and likely levels of take-up. Such projections are hard to make and can be wide of the mark. The severe disability premium in income support and housing benefit was introduced in 1988 on the basis that it was unlikely that more than 10,000 people would be entitled. By 1993 there were 131,000 recipients, an unexpected expense for a government trying to curb social security expenditure. Disability working allowance, on the other hand, introduced in 1992 with an expectation of attracting some 50,000 recipients, appeared to have a take-up rate of only 17 per cent by autumn 1993 (Rowlingson and Berthoud, 1994) and by January 1995 there were still only just over 5,000 recipients (DSS, 1995c). Those who plan overall social security expenditure and prioritise resources have a strong interest in the development of techniques of measurement and quantification of eligibility and take-up.

Finally, the take-up measure has been seen as an indicator of social justice. Van Oorschot (1991) argues that people's eligibility for a benefit defines their insufficient share of resources to which they have rights. If non-take-up means that people are deprived of their rights and entitlements, then they are subject to social injustice. The discourse of social justice is rarely used within current British social security policymaking. The idea that the social security system is an institution for promoting just distribution of resources does not fit well with more recent policy emphases on consumerism, choice and individual responsibility (Taylor-Gooby, 1994). This does not mean that we should discount this aspect of the importance of take-up.

Having looked at what the terms take-up and non-take-up mean, and why these concepts are so important, the next section considers how such estimates are derived.

Measuring take-up

Government estimates of take-up of income-related benefits have traditionally used a mix of data from administrative records from the Department of Social Security and local authority housing benefit departments, together with survey data from continuous household surveys of income and expenditure. Clearly, the actual numbers of recipients and the amount of money received are available from administrative records. It is counting the eligible people with apparent entitlements which they are not receiving which presents a greater challenge. The only real test of eligibility of a non-recipient is by submission of an application, to see what decision is made by the actual administrator of the benefit. This is sometimes tried in small-scale studies (for example, Corden and Craig, 1991; McKay and Marsh, 1994) but for official national estimates, eligibility of survey respondents is 'modelled' on the basis of information they provide about their personal and financial circumstances.

The key data source for the official estimates is now the Family Resources Survey (FRS) a continuous household survey reaching around 26,000 households each year. In previous years government statisticians used the Family Expenditure Survey (FES), but the FRS now provides a much larger sample, improving the reliability of the estimates by reduction in sampling error. The FRS does not, however, contain sufficient information about incomes of self-employed people to allow take-up estimates to be made for this group, nor are people living outside private households included, for example those living in residential care and nursing homes, and in bed and breakfast accommodation.

For income support, housing benefit and council tax benefit estimates are now presented as ranges, between which it can be assumed the true take-up lies (DSS, 1997). This is a recent development. Earlier measures were presented as 'point estimates' (see, for example, DSS, 1993) but there is now greater understanding of the possible extent of bias in the baseline or point estimates, which are now used as only the first stage in the calculation. For income support, housing benefit and council tax benefit the formulae used in this first stage, to set baseline estimates of take-up are as follows:

$$\text{caseload take-up} = \frac{R_{admin}}{R_{admin} + ENR_{FRS}}$$

$$\text{expenditure take-up} = \frac{R_{admin} \times \pounds R_{admin}}{(R_{admin} \times \pounds R_{admin}) + (ENR_{FRS} \times \pounds ENR_{FRS})}$$

where R represents the number of recipients
ENR represents the number of entitled non-recipients
subscripts refer to the data source
$\pounds$R represents the average weekly amount received by recipients
$\pounds$ENR represents the average weekly amount unclaimed by entitled non-recipients.

The next step for the statisticians is to assess the extent of bias. Various sources of error can distort the baseline estimates of case-load take-up. Respondents may misreport their receipt or non-receipt, for example, it is not unusual for pensioners to report a 'retirement pension' which actually includes small income support top-ups. Some payments may be going to people with no entitlement, for example as a result of processing delay or administrative error. At the level of analysis, calculations from the data available may not identify true entitlement or non-entitlement. Again, at the analytical level, multiplications from the sample counts to reflect the true numbers and characteristics of relevant people in the overall population, a process known as 'grossing-up', may be inaccurate. In moving from base-line estimates to take-up ranges the analyst uses statistical techniques to estimate upper and lower limits for the different sources of error, and assesses how these errors interact. This is done separately for each benefit, and each family and tenure type.

Family credit estimates are further complicated by the fact that, once awarded, family credit remains in payment for six months regardless of changes in circumstances. This means that it is not sufficient to compare people's current circumstances of work or income and their receipt or non-receipt of family credit with the current eligibility criteria for this benefit. Further adjustments are necessary. It is not possible to go on to produce error ranges, thus the baseline estimates are the most accurate that can be achieved for family credit.

There has been considerable development in government's expertise in take-up estimation during the last few years, and readers with a special interest can follow the story from the Department of Social Security's own publications (DSS, 1991; 1994; 1995a; 1995b; 1997). It is important to know how the official figures are produced, but these are not the only way of producing take-up estimates. The government estimate outlined above gives the proportion of measured eligible recipients among the sum of measured recipients and eligible non-recipients. An alternative estimate, favoured by econometricians such as Fry and Stark (1993), gives the proportion of eligible recipients among all eligible people. Duclos (1992) suggests two other ways of making an estimate, both of which may be calculated from survey data alone. The details of these alternative measures are not spelled out in this chapter, but when reading research findings about levels of take-up it is important to consider what kind of measure was being used.

Take-up estimates of a different order to those based on national surveys and administrative records are the 'snap-shot' counts conducted by researchers working at a local level or focusing on groups of people with special characteristics. Researchers use their own, sometimes detailed, knowledge of social security rules and how these are administered to decide the entitlement status of respondents in specially designed surveys (for example, Marsh and McKay, 1993) or people interviewed in depth (Corden and Craig, 1991). The first stage in many local welfare rights campaigns has been a demonstration of apparently low take-up of particular benefits in an area or among a particular group of people, and developments in the field of hand-held computers have provided new opportunities here for 'screening' people and investigating levels of take-up of benefits. Such smaller-scale initiatives have proved useful and informative, and have been specially valuable in focusing attention on issues to do with the take-up of those benefits for which no official take-up estimates are presented.

It is worth emphasising again, however, that the only real test of eligibility is submission of an application. Drawing on experience of recontacting apparently eligible non-claimants of family credit, some of whom had indeed submitted an application, McKay and Marsh (1995) concluded that some of the elements of eligibility for a benefit such as family credit are so complex and unstable that eligibility itself is an unstable state. They observed that 'the more you learn about eligible non-claimants, the less eligible they become' (ibid., p. 5), a lesson that this author had also learned from many years' research on the family credit population. The point is that although there is much to learn from attempting to measure take-up, across a range of benefits, such quantification remains inexact and provides only a partial view of access to benefits.

Useful new perspectives come from work done by Walker and colleagues (Vincent *et al.*, 1991; Walker with Ashworth, 1994). They suggest that there are temporal aspects of targeting and administration of benefits that must be considered in evaluating take-up rates, and that some benefits, by nature of their structure and design, can be expected to have lower achievable take-up rates than others. Features that are likely to be important here include the structure and eligibility criteria of the benefit, the way in which duration of award is linked to changing circumstances over time, and the length of time the benefit has been operating. We might expect, they argue, that a new benefit, with relatively short duration of award and targeted at a volatile population will have a lower attainable take-up rate than a benefit which, once awarded, lasts a relatively long time. Pursuing this argument suggests that take-up rates for income support for families with children are unlikely ever to attain the level of take-up of child benefit by such families, and makes us think harder about what an 'acceptable' take-up rate might be, and whether new benefits should be introduced which, as a result of structural design, are likely always to have relatively low take-up rates. This is discussed further in the following section.

Understanding how take-up is quantified and what the different kinds of measures of non-take-up mean we can move to one of the most persistent puzzles in social policy – why do so many people fail to receive so much money to which they are entitled?

Reasons for non-take-up

The government's estimates of the possible range of non-take-up suggest that between £1,210 million and £1,870 million of income support went unclaimed in 1995–96 (DSS, 1997). A further £300 million family credit apparently went unclaimed by parents with low earnings, and unclaimed housing benefit that could have helped towards people's rent may have been as much as £760 million. There is probably still much to learn about why this happens. This section of the chapter reviews what is known now, and explains how such understanding has developed.

Interest in the reasons for non-take-up of benefits arose as a 'by-product' of research on poverty during the 1950s and early 1960s (Craig, 1991) and the association of non-take-up with impoverishment and low living standards has continued to draw attention. During the 1970s a number of new income-related benefits were introduced, along with new benefits to help meet the extra costs of disability and caring. This brought new groups of people with special financial needs into focus, and the 1970s saw the development of widespread welfare rights activity, as advocates and campaigning groups realised the scope for improving people's standard of living by ensuring their full take-up of the resources available (Alcock and Shepherd, 1987).

Most of the research on take-up during the 1970s was conducted at a local level, the chief concern being to identify ways in which deterrents to claiming might be overcome (see Corden, 1983 and Craig, 1991 for reviews). People who were asked directly about their delayed claims or non-claiming behaviour often explained that they had not known earlier about their entitlement, that feelings of pride prevented their coming forward, or they had not been able to cope with the process of administration. The general view emerged that non-take-up could be attributed to three main factors: ignorance, stigma and administrative complexity (Deacon and Bradshaw, 1983), and that these factors inter-acted. For example, providing advice and information often still did not trigger applications from people who said that the main reason for not claiming had been lack of knowledge. It proved hard to increase and maintain take-up levels, and despite some understanding of possible deterrents to claiming, by the end of the 1970s the picture was still one of general frustration and lack of clarity.

In retrospect, Craig talks of this period as one of 'conceptual clutter' (1991, p. 544) which was ripe for a breakthrough of new ideas. These came in the early 1980s in the form of new 'models' of the claiming process, based on psychological and attitudinal theory. The most influential models were Kerr's 'threshold model' (1982; 1983) which he developed to investigate the differential take-up of supplementary pension, and Ritchie and Matthews' 'trade-off model' used in a study of rent allowances (1982).

The Kerr model

Kerr was a psychologist who was intrigued by the question of why some retirement pensioners were not claiming the supplementary pension due to them. Interviews with elderly people led Kerr to present the claiming process as passage through a series of six constructs. These are the six necessary conditions of claiming which, together, are sufficient to bring about a claim. He suggested that the six constructs must be passed in a determinate sequence and the first threshold 'unachieved' prevents a claim, as represented in Figure 6.1.

In simple terms, according to this model, an elderly person who would have liked to have more money; knew that there were supplementary pensions and how to make the first contact with the administrative office; thought she might be eligible; considered that even a little extra each week would be worth having; held the view that she had as much right to this money as anybody else and, finally, knew that her financial situation was not going to improve otherwise, would make a claim. Her neighbour, in similar financial circumstances and with the same understanding of the availability of the supplementary pension, but who could not bring herself to ask for help, failed to reach the threshold of beliefs and feelings necessary, and failed to claim.

Kerr's model represented a major breakthrough in conceptual approaches to take-up and has been highly influential. Elements of the model have been incorporated into several subsequent research studies, (for example Corden, 1983; 1987; Davies and Ritchie, 1988; Graham, 1984; Millar and Cooke, 1984). Current feeling is that Kerr's constructs remain of great heuristic value, but there are a number of shortcomings to the model. It has not been subject to much testing, largely because the prospective design required would be costly and hard to conduct. The sequentiality of the thresholds does not seem to hold up, in some studies, and it seems that strong beliefs or attitudes on some constructs can balance out or over-rule the weak beliefs or negative attitudes on other constructs which would have been expected to stop the claiming

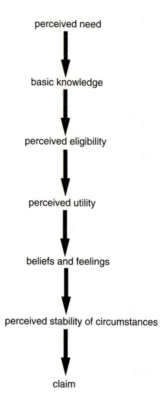

Figure 6.1   Kerr's model of claiming behaviour

process. The model does not easily accommodate the interactions between household members that are known to be important, and does not accommodate administrative effects on the outcomes of claiming. The model seems to miss some important factors noted by other researchers, such as the effect of certain 'triggers' in precipitating applications. Both Corden (1983) and Graham (1984) noted that long delays in claiming were often brought to an end by a trigger such as a new piece of information or a sudden need-related event.

Craig (1991) and van Oorschot (1995) discuss fully the main disadvantages of Kerr's model, while acknowledging the value of Kerr's original ideas. The second most influential model of the claiming process during the 1980s was that developed by Ritchie and Matthews, to which we now turn.

The Ritchie and Matthews model

Ritchie and Matthews (1982) were working on their own model of claiming behaviour at the same time as Kerr was developing his. They compared claimants and non-claimants of rent allowances for private tenants, and found that perceptions of need and eligibility were critical. They thought the most useful representation of factors determining the claiming decision was that of a process of reconciliation of opposing influences, using the notion of 'trade-off'. Although less well known than the Kerr model, Ritchie and Matthews' approach introduced valuable ideas such as the effective intervention of other people in encouraging applications, and the complex roots of perceptions of eligibility.

Further discussion of the 'modelling' approach that was so influential in take-up research throughout the 1980s can be found in Craig's review (1991). The alternative to asking people about their attitudes and comparing this with their claiming behaviour is to use data from household surveys to investigate the relationship between observed variables and probabilities of claiming. This is called the econometric approach, and was the second main stream of research on take-up during the 1980s.

The econometric approach

A number of studies to estimate and offer some explanations for non-take-up have been conducted by economists, using statistical techniques on large data sets and applying economic cost-benefit rational choice models. The idea is to assess the explanatory power of the costs or 'disutilities' to claiming which, in this context, include non-monetary components such as stigma and information costs. The problem here is that the data sets used, such as the FES, do not include variables that indicate directly the kinds of costs involved. It is necessary to use proxy variables, which leave findings open to a number of interpretations. The economic approaches are probably most useful when the statistical findings are considered alongside results from more direct behavioural or attitudinal investigation, pointing to issues and areas where specially designed surveys or small-scale investigations might be most fruitful.

For example, when Dorsett and Heady (1991) looked at the take-up of family income supplement and housing benefit over the period 1984–87, using FES data, one intriguing result was that people with large housing benefit entitlements were more likely to take up not only housing benefit but also family income supplement. One suggestion offered for this one-way effect was that people tended to discover family income supplement while claiming housing benefit. Another suggestion was that large housing benefit entitlements may be better indicators of 'need' than family income supplement entitlements, such that take-up was associated more with 'the push' of poverty than the 'pull' of the value of entitlements.

There are fairly consistent findings from this kind of research that the probability of claiming income-related benefits increases as the level of entitlement increases (Blundell *et al.*, 1988; Fry and Stark, 1993) and that if the level of entitlement is held constant, the probability of claiming decreases as income rises. Again, different interpretations are possible, as van Oorschot points out (1995). It might be the case that people trade off the costs and revenues: so it seems more worthwhile spending time and effort to get a larger amount of money, or it seems less worthwhile to go to the trouble, anyway, to people who are financially less pressed. It might be, however, that people with very small entitlements are less certain about their eligibility, being right at the boundary of entitlement and are more likely to make the wrong decision that they are not entitled, and hence, that there is no point applying. A third suggestion is that there may be effects of administrative error (Duclos, 1995). For example, a person near the boundary of eligibility, with a small entitlement of £2 may be more likely to be assessed as ineligible than a person with a large entitlement of £25 as a result of a small error in assessment of entitlement. These are all areas worth looking at in greater depth, using appropriate techniques.

Craig's review of research on take-up (1991) presents further examples of econometric studies including work conducted in USA, and van Oorschot (1995) adds more recent material. There is no doubt that the intensity of research on this topic during the 1980s pushed forward our understanding of the issues involved. This, in turn, made possible some developments in promotional and advertising strategies, and administrative improvements such as better designed forms and easier telephone access which did have some effect in gradually improving take-up of benefits such as family credit.

However, Craig (1991) was uncertain about the value of pursuing current research approaches much further. He wrote: 'As understanding of the claiming process improves, the methodological constraints get tighter' (ibid., p. 562). At the same time, new criticisms of the current conceptual approach to take-up began to arise. McLaughlin *et al.* observed that 'an essentially pragmatic approach towards take-up (what can be done to ameliorate low take-up) has developed' (1990, p. 1). This narrow approach, they argued, had led to unsuccessful claiming by ineligible people being almost completely ignored, although this was as common, if not more so, as delayed take-up or non-claiming by eligible people and led to costly inefficiencies in the administrative arrangements. It became hard to fit new benefits such as the social fund into traditional concepts and measures of take-up (Huby and Whyley, 1996). The stage was set for another new breakthrough.

Interestingly, it has been a comparative approach that has been useful in opening up two new streams of work which, together, are changing perspectives on take-up. Van Oorschot, working in the Netherlands, developed some of his ideas from an international review of take-up research, and Walker, in Britain, had been interested in results of longitudinal research from the USA. The following section of the chapter looks at these two approaches which are taking us towards a new 'generation' of take-up research for the 1990s.

Van Oorschot's interactive model of multi-level influences

From their international review of research on non-take-up, van Oorschot and Kolkhuis Tancke (research summarised in English by van Oorschot, 1991) suggested that benefits which showed high levels of non-take-up tended to share some characteristics. There were structural features of benefit design or administration, they argued, which led to greater probabilities of non-take-up. The influence of these structural features meant that it was not enough to try to understand take-up and non-take-up only in terms of client decision-making and behaviour. Drawing on these ideas van Oorschot went on to develop an interactive model of the three levels of influence, represented in Figure 6.2.

Factors influencing take-up operate at three interactive levels: the benefit scheme, the administrative arrangements and the population in scope. There are thus three groups of 'actors': policy-makers, administrators and clients.

Policy-makers determine the rules of the benefit and how it is to be allocated, the budget available and where responsibility lies for administrative arrangements. They set the legal context and the organisational framework. At this level of influence, van Oorschot argues, non-take-up is likely to be higher in schemes that:

- have a high density of rules and guidelines;
- contain complex rules;
- contain vague criteria of entitlement;

- contain a means test;
- are aimed at groups in society who are the subject of negative valuation (associated with negative prejudices);
- supplement other sources of income;
- leave the initiative to start the claiming process fully to the applicant.

Reviewing the British research literature leads Corden (1995) to suggest that there may be additional structural features that tend to contribute to non-take-up by eligible people, for example:

- a test of disability;
- overlap or interaction with other benefits;
- challenge to cultural norms or characteristics.

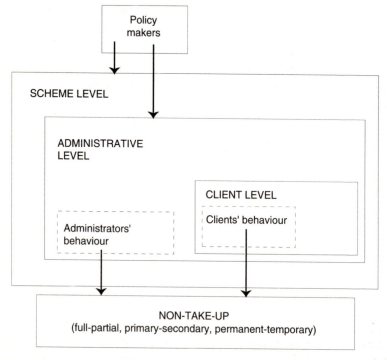

Figure 6.2   An interactive model of the multi-level influences on non-take-up
Source: van Oorschot (1996, p. 11).

The second level of influence, according to van Oorschot's model, is the administrative level. It is administrators who communicate with clients, put the rules into operation and make decisions about entitlement, affecting take-up directly (for example, in adjudication of claims) or indirectly (in their effect on clients' claiming behaviour). Corden (1995) looks at recent research on take-up under headings which fit this second level of influence:

- information supply;
- service provision;
- application forms;
- subsequent negotiations;
- administrative links between benefits;
- accuracy in decision-making;
- policing the system.

The strength of van Oorschot's model is that it gives equal weight to structural features of design and administration, alongside aspects of client behaviour, and offers a more useful perspective on the whole claiming process. It allows incorporation of features such as administrative error, and information supply, and tips the balance of perceived responsibilities for achieving take-up back towards policy-makers and administrators, rather than seeking explanations for non-take-up in terms of the ignorance or irrationality of clients. Recently, Huby and Whyley (1996) have endorsed this interactive model as a more useful framework than that of Kerr for conceptualisation and analysis of take-up of the social fund, a discretionary benefit.

Within this interactive model, van Oorschot attempted to refine conceptualisation of the claiming decisions made by the client, using findings from cross-sectional surveys of households in two cities in the Netherlands (van Oorschot, 1995). He argued that once the basic knowledge and perceived eligibility thresholds had been achieved, the most important part of the process, then the rest of the decision-making process represented an overall trade-off between factors that promoted and deterred claiming. 'Triggers', especially in the form of information or a newly perceived need, could be important catalysts to action, either prompting claims or altering the balance in the trade-off. There is an overall emphasis on understanding take-up as a dynamic process, with movement at all three levels of the model, and reaction and interaction of the different actors.

A focus on the dynamics of populations in scope for benefits, and temporal aspects of benefit receipt tells us even more about whether the appropriate people are receiving what is due to them. In the final section of the chapter, we look at what might be learned about take-up by paying attention to the dimension of time.

Dynamic aspects of take-up

We have really only just begun to understand how important temporal aspects may be in framing social security analysis. Some of the early ideas have been formulated by Walker (1994; 1996) and we illustrate these by describing a new perspective on the take-up measure, and then, the idea that there may be different 'attainable take-up rates' for different benefits.

First, the reliability of a take-up measure based on point-in-time estimates is likely to be reduced if the dynamics of the eligible population are different from those of the population in receipt. Walker describes findings from longitudinal research on the US Food Stamp programme (Carr, *et al.*, 1984) showing that turnover was greater among households who were eligible than among those who actually claimed food stamps. As a result, take-up measures based on point-in-time counts may overestimate take-up: the denominator of the take-up fraction excludes disproportionate numbers of households who are eligible for only a short time. Walker suggests that this effect may be generalisable to other benefits.

There may be a similar effect as a result of dynamics in the benefit structure. Current eligibility of self-employed people for benefits such as housing benefit, family credit and income support may depend on historical measures of income which do not match current profitability (Boden and Corden, 1994). The resultant situations of individual self-employed people may thus be highly complex, in terms of traditional take-up concepts, and the financial information necessary to resolve matters may be unmanageable in the context of take-up research. Self-employed people are generally excluded from official take-up measures, although in 1994 self-employed people represented some 13 per cent of all those in paid work (Corden, 1996). Having an official take-up measure which systematically excludes such a proportion of the population is rarely questioned. However, recent growth in the numbers of self-employed people and their heavy representation among low income groups suggest that we may now need new ways of evaluating outcome of benefit allocation, to stand alongside more traditional estimates.

A second issue arising from dynamic interactions between the claimant population and benefit structure is the likelihood of there being different 'attainable take-up' levels for different benefits. We might expect a lower attainable take-up rate, say, for income support which has a relatively short duration of award but is targeted at a volatile population, than for child benefit, which, once awarded, lasts many years with few opportunities for becoming an eligible non-claimant. Other temporal aspects which might be important include the length of time a benefit has been operating. Low take-up rates and high levels of applications from ineligible people are both aspects likely to be associated with relatively new benefits – time is needed for diffusion of correct information and correction of misinformation.

Policy response and the way forward

As a study in the way knowledge develops, the 'take-up story' is a fascinating one. The energy with which the topic has been pursued continuously for more than three decades has been fuelled from various sources: the frustration of the persistence of poverty against a background of apparently massive underclaiming of entitlements; the attraction of trying to understand human behaviour that at first sight may seem irrational or even self-destructive; the desperation of governments committed to targeting when confronted with such apparent lack of success. We see distinct stages in the development of ideas, and the influence here of some of the main sponsors of research. For governments have been primarily interested in why apparently ineligible people do not claim their due, and, since the mid-1980s, the need to control social security spending and reduce unemployment have acted together to focus government interest even more narrowly, on the non-take-up of income-related benefits that maintain work incentives. Little attention has ever been paid to what might be considered just as interesting and important – why do so many people apply for benefits for which they are not entitled, causing, in turn, massive administrative expense and inefficiency, and apparent human disappointment and frustration?

The influence of sponsorship of research may also be one of the reasons for the concentration of studies based on attempts to model claimant behaviour. The author has suggested (1995) that such models are based firmly within the ideology of individualism, and recent governments have tended to be most interested in models of the claiming process that did not challenge predominant ideology. It is interesting that the recent major contribution to understanding, that gives equal status to aspects of design and structure as to claimant decision-making, has come from outside Britain. There have, of course, been many valuable local studies on take-up in this country, including research on disability benefits, which have emphasised the importance of structural factors, but in terms of developing policy, government has tended to favour findings from research directly commissioned. This chapter has not attempted to do justice to the wealth of research on take-up conducted by welfare rights organisations, agencies and organisations representing disabled people and their carers, local authorities or health services. Reviews of this important work may be read elsewhere (for example Alcock and Shepherd, 1987; Falkingham, 1985).

Apart from looking at take-up in terms of a story of the development of knowledge, how much of what has been learned has been applied in the policy process? It is quite hard to make a strong argument that much of our understanding has been rapidly applied, with major impact. Certainly, policy-makers have responded quickly to some of the pointers to adjustments or improvements in administrative procedure which might be expected to influence take-up of income-related benefits. There have been major initiatives to improve access for claimants to the administrative system, for example telephone services, the design of forms and standard letters, the environment of local offices, 'fast tracking' applications from some people who might be expected to have special needs. Attention has been paid to rules and procedures for self-employed people. There have been major efforts to improve services for people from ethnic minorities (see Chapter 9), and some disabled people, for example those with sensory impairments (see Chapter 7). There is continuous selective advertising and promotional activity. In the case of family credit, there would appear to be some success. The most recent take-up estimates do compare favourably with previously disappointing results. Similarly, the take-up of income support by families with children does show some improvement over recent years, on a more moderate scale. Among other groups of people, however, such as pensioners, take-up of income support seems to remain hard to budge.

The most recent developments in take-up research now present a real challenge to government policy. If it is true that attainable rates for income-related benefits are likely to remain depressed by structural features, what does this tell us about a policy firmly committed to increasingly selective targeting? It suggests that some targets will remain hard to hit with accuracy, despite intensive expensive administrative efforts, and receptivity and compliance of the population in scope. It means acceptance of the fact that proportions of people who are defined as having entitlements to a greater share in the country's resources are almost certain not to receive them. If van Oorschot's emphasis on structure and administration is widely adopted in understanding the take-up of benefits, it seems inconceivable that another benefit like the new disability working allowance could be introduced in the belief that this would be a generally useful and efficient way of allocating resources. Early evaluation of this new income-related benefit, which incorporates almost every one of the structural design features which van Oorschot and Corden suggest are likely to be associated with low take-up, produced a take-up estimate of 17 per cent (Rowlingson and Berthoud, 1994).

It is hard to see in which direction 'the take-up story' will go now. When latest research findings point so strongly away from a policy committed to more selective targeting there may be less government interest in sponsoring further work. It is also true that full take-up of income-related benefits would inflate social security expenditure by a significant amount, at a time when policy-makers are trying to reduce the bill. Research commissioned from outside government, and more research coming from abroad, will apply different contexts and set new agendas. Those who have followed avidly the 'take-up story' do not know whether they have now come to the last page, or have just read the introduction to the next instalment.

References

Alcock, P. and Shepherd, J. (1987) 'Take-up campaigns: fighting poverty through the post', *Critical Social Policy* 19: 52–67.

Blundell, R., Fry, V. and Walker, I. (1988) 'Modelling the take-up of means-tested benefits: the case of housing benefits in the UK', *Economic Journal* 98: 58–94.

Boden, R. and Corden, A. (1994) *Measuring Low Incomes: Self-Employment and Family Credit*, London: HMSO.

Callender, C., Court, G., Thompson, M. and Patch, A. (1994) *Employers and Family Credit*, Department of Social Security Research Report No. 32, London: HMSO.

Carr, T., Doyle, P. and Lubitz, I. (1984) *Turnover in Food Stamp Participation*, Washington, DC: Mathematica Policy Research, prepared for US Department of Agriculture, Food and Nutrition Service.

Corden, A. (1983) *Taking Up a Means-Tested Benefit: The Process of Claiming Family Income Supplement*, London: HMSO.

—— (1987) *Disappointed Applicants. A Study of Unsuccessful Claims for Family Income Supplement*, Aldershot: Avebury.

—— (1995) *Changing Perspectives on Benefit Take-Up*, London: HMSO.

—— (1996) 'Enterprising claimants? Self-employed people and benefit take-up in Great Britain', in W. van Oorschot (ed.) *New Perspectives on the Non-Take-Up of Social Security Benefits*, Netherlands: Tilburg University Press.

Corden, A. and Craig, P. (1991) *Perceptions of Family Credit*, London: HMSO.

Craig, P. (1991) 'Costs and benefits: a review of research on take-up of income-related benefits', *Journal of Social Policy* 20(4): 537–566.

Davies, C. and Ritchie, J. (1988) *Tipping the Balance: A Study of Non-Take-Up of Benefits in an Inner City Area*, London: HMSO.

Deacon, A. and Bradshaw, J. (1983) *Reserved for the Poor: The Means Test in British Social Policy*, Oxford: Blackwell and Robertson.

DHSS (1985) *Reform of Social Security: Programme for Action*, Department of Social Security, White Paper, Cmnd 9691, London: HMSO.

Dorsett, R. and Heady, C. (1991) 'The take-up of means-tested benefits by working families with children', *Fiscal Studies* 12(4): 22–32.

DSS (1991) *Income Related Benefits: Estimates of Take-up in 1987*, Technical Notes, Analytical Services Division, London: Department of Social Security.

—— (1993) *Income Related Benefits: Estimates of Take-up in 1989*, Analytical Services Division, London: Department of Social Security.

—— (1994) *Income Related Benefits: Estimates of Take-Up in 1990 and 1991*, London: Department of Social Security.

—— (1995a) *Income Related Benefits: Estimates of Take-Up in 1992*, London: Department of Social Security.

—— (1995b) *Income Related Benefits: Estimates of Take-Up in 1993/94*, London: Department of Social Security.

—— (1995c) *Social Security Statistics, 1995*, London: Department of Social Security.

—— (1997) *Income Related Benefits: Estimates of Take-Up in 1995/96*, London: Department of Social Security

Duclos, J-Y. (1992) *The Take-Up of State Benefits: An Application to Supplementary Benefits in Britain Using the FES*, Discussion Paper WSP/71, STICERD, London: London School of Economics.

—— (1995) 'Modelling the take-up of state support', *Journal of Public Economics* 58: 391–415.

Eardley, T. and Corden, A. (1996) *Low Income Self-Employment: Work, Benefits and Living Standards*, Aldershot: Avebury.

Falkingham, F. (1985) *Take-up of Benefit: A Literature Review*, Nottingham: Benefits Research Unit, University of Nottingham.

Fry, V. and Stark, G. (1993) *The Take-Up of Means-Tested Benefits, 1984–90*, London: Institute of Fiscal Studies.

Graham, J. (1984) *Take-up of Family Income Supplement: Knowledge, Attitudes and Experience – Claimants and Non-Claimants*, Occasional Paper No. 2, Belfast: Policy Planning and Research Unit.

Huby, M. and Whyley, C. (1996) 'Take-up and the Social Fund', *Journal of Social Policy* 25(1): 1–18.

Kerr, S. (1982) 'Deciding about supplementary pensions: a provisional model', *Journal of Social Policy* 11(4): 505–17.

—— (1983) *Making Ends Meet: An Investigation into the Non-Claiming of Supplementary Pensions*, London: Bedford Square Press.

Marsh, A. and McKay, S. (1993) *Families, Work and Benefits*, London: Policy Studies Institute.

McKay, S. and Marsh, A. (1995) *Why Didn't They Claim?*, London: Policy Studies Institute.

McLaughlin, E., Ritchie, J. and Walker, R. (1990) 'The claiming of social security benefits', paper presented to IRISS Conference 1990, Social Policy Research Unit, University of York.

Millar, J. and Cooke, K. (1984) *A Study of the Take-up of One Parent Benefit in Hackney*, DHSS 227, Social Policy Research Unit Working Paper, York: University of York.

Noble, M., Smith, G. and Munby, T. (1992) *The Take-up of Family Credit*, Department of Applied Social Studies and Social Research, Oxford: University of Oxford.

Oorschot, W. van (1991) 'Non-take-up of social security benefits in Europe', *Journal of European Social Policy* 1(1): 15–30.

—— (1995) *Realizing Rights*, Aldershot: Avebury.

—— (1996) 'Modelling non-take-up', in W. van Oorschot (ed.) *New Perspectives on the Non-Take-Up of Social Security Benefits*, Netherlands: Tilburg University Press.

Ritchie, J. and Matthews, A. (1982) *Take-up of Rent Allowances: An In-Depth Study*, London: Social and Community Planning Research.

Rowlingson, K. and Berthoud, R. (1994) *Evaluating the Disability Working Allowance: First Findings*, London: Policy Studies Institute.

Taylor-Gooby, P. (1994) 'Post-modernism and social policy: a great leap backwards?' *Journal of Social Policy* 23(3): 385–404.

Walker, R. (1996) 'Benefit dynamics, targeting and take-up', in W. van Oorschot (ed.) *New Perspectives on the Non-Take-up of Social Security Benefits*, Netherlands: Tilburg University Press.

Walker, R. with Ashworth, K. (1994) *Poverty Dynamics: Issues and Examples*, Aldershot: Avebury.

Vincent, J., Ashworth, K. and Walker, R. (1991) *Taking Account of Time in the Targeting and Administration of Benefits*, Discussion Paper 141, Centre for Research in Social Policy, Loughborough University of Technology.

7 Social security, poverty and disability

Helen Barnes and Sally Baldwin

Disability is likely to result in poverty not only for disabled individuals but for their wider families. Is this a 'natural' consequence of inability to work or the result of discriminatory policies and practice? Does social security policy alleviate or create poverty? This chapter aims to examine the causes of poverty for disabled people, and to assess the types of policies adopted.

One immediate difficulty when discussing 'disability' is that a great deal of confusion, and controversy, arises over the language used to describe it. As Martin *et al.* (1988) acknowledge, terms are used inconsistently in a wide range of contexts, from legislation and research to medicine and everyday conversation. Often, different terms are used to refer to identical concepts; while the same term (for example 'disability' itself) is used to describe quite different concepts. Moreover, many administrative systems for assessing disability, in order to decide eligibility for benefits of one kind or another, seek to distinguish between 'disabled' and 'non-disabled' people, whereas disability is more usefully viewed as a continuum. At the heart of disputes about correct terms lies a much deeper dispute about the meaning of disability and the cause of the disadvantage with which it is commonly associated. These disputes are too complex to pursue in any detail here. Essentially, however, what is at issue is whether 'disability' is best regarded as the outcome of an impairment (physical or mental) as a disadvantage created by society, or some mix of these.

Until the early 1980s the first view prevailed. A major breakthrough was provided by the World Health Organisation classification published in that year. This distinguishes three separate concepts:

1   *Impairment:* 'Any loss or abnormality of psychological, physiological or anatomical structure or function.' In other words, parts or systems of the body do not work correctly.

2   *Disability*: 'Any restriction or lack (resulting from an impairment) of ability to perform an activity in the manner or within the range considered normal for a human being.' This refers to things which people cannot do because of an impairment.

3   *Handicap*: 'A disadvantage for a given individual, resulting from an impairment or disability, that limits or prevents the fulfilment of a social role for that individual.' This refers to the relationship between the person and others and the limitations that follow from not being able to do certain things.

(Wood, 1981)

The classification was regarded by many as a major advance in clarity; the conceptual distinction between disability and handicap was perceived as particularly useful. However, disabled activists and scholars object to the fact that this classification still regards 'handicap' as a natural outcome of physical limitations. The restrictions experienced by people with impairments are, they argue, the result of particular *social* arrangements (Oliver, 1990). What has become known as 'the social model of disability' is based on a simple twofold classification:

1   *Impairment*: Lacking all or part of a limb, or having a defective limb, organism or mechanism of the body.

2   *Disability*: The disadvantage or restriction of social activity caused by a contemporary social organisation which takes no or little account of people who have physical impairments and thus excludes them from the mainstream of social activities.

(Union of the Physically Impaired Against Segregation, 1976)

This debate continues to unfold and recent work by disabled writers seeks to refine the social model of disability to take account of intrinsic features of impairment, such as pain and fatigue, which may limit what people can do, regardless of how social arrangements are arranged and adjusted (Crow, 1992; French, 1993; Morris, 1992). Space does not permit a discussion of the extensive literature on this issue. It is, however, important to bear in mind that most of the research reviewed in this chapter uses some form of the WHO classification, or is strongly influenced by its approach. Administrative systems based on the social model of disability have yet to be developed.

Thus, the major surveys of disability in Britain, carried out in 1976 by the Office of Population Censuses and Surveys (OPCS), defined disability by reference to self-reported restrictions in activities of daily living. This was further developed to create a sophisticated, ten point, scale, to measure the severity of disability (Martin *et al.*, 1988). This survey made no attempt to assess how far social arrangements, such as the built environment or employers' recruitment policies, made the *effect* of an impairment more or less severe (Abberley, 1992; Oliver, 1990). The OPCS figures are, however, thus subject to caveats. Nevertheless, they provide extremely valuable information on the prevalence and impact of disability in Britain.

According to the OPCS definition, there are around six million disabled people in Britain, of whom about a third are of working age. The vast majority live in private households, although around 7 per cent live in communal establishments such as hostels, hospitals or residential care homes. Contrary to popular stereotypes, the vast majority of disabled people are older people (69 per cent are aged over 60), often with chronic illnesses, who may or may not define themselves as disabled (Martin *et al.*, 1988). Severity of disability increases with age. Almost half of people in the highest severity category living in private households are aged over 75. The main impairments these people iden- tify as causes of disability are musculo-skeletal complaints,[1] which were mentioned by 46 per cent of respondents. Ear complaints (mentioned by 38 per cent) and eye complaints (by 22 per cent) were also signifi- cant.[2] For those living in communal establishments, mental health problems or learning difficulties were the main cause of disability, affecting half of all residents, while a third had musculo-skeletal prob- lems (ibid., 1988).

The 1980s and 1990s have seen disabled people achieve an unprece- dented political visibility. An increasingly self-confident and vocal movement of disabled people has identified disability as a civil rights issue, campaigned for legislative protection, and won the support of the general public (Gooding, 1994). Government hostility to the civil rights project, due largely to anticipated effects on public expenditure, has prevented any of the bills introduced from becoming law. However, the process has proved so politically damaging that the government was obliged to issue its own, more limited, proposals for legislation in July 1994. The Disability Discrimination Act, which became law on 8 November 1995, forbids discrimination in the field of employment, and in the provision of goods and services, subject to protective clauses which limit the amount of costs which employers and other agencies will be expected to bear (see Doyle, 1995, for a detailed analysis of the new Act). Crucially, however, it provides no specific, enforceable, rights in the areas of education and transport.

These recent, and limited, advances seem unlikely to change the fact that the majority of disabled people in the United Kingdom live in poverty. They are excluded from participation in the ordinary life of the community not only by physical and attitudinal barriers, but by low incomes which make it difficult to enjoy normal activities like having a holiday or buying new clothes. Their poverty is the result of a lack of rights – to employment, to adequate incomes when unable to work, to personal assistance. It is also likely to hinder them in the exercise of those rights which they do possess.

Disability and the risk of poverty

Disabled people account for a small proportion of the total population of people with very low incomes compared, for instance, to families with children. However, unlike families with children, the great majority of disabled people have very low incomes – disability greatly increases the probability of becoming poor. Layard *et al.* (1978), using a poverty scale of 120 per cent of Supplementary Benefit (a less generous measure than the 140 per cent generally used) found that over half of families with a permanently disabled head of household had incomes below this level. The OPCS surveys found similar results.[3] Among households containing a disabled person of working age, 73 per cent had incomes below the median level for the general population. Moreover, 34 per cent had incomes less than half the median, as compared to 23 per cent of all non-pensioner households (Martin and White, 1988). Berthoud (1993) re-analysed the OPCS data using the long-term rate of Supplementary Benefit as a 'base' poverty line. According to this analysis, 18 per cent of disabled people were in poverty. When the measure was adjusted to take account of the additional costs of disability (see below), this figure rose to 45 per cent of disabled people. Only 13 per cent achieved the 'prosperity' standard of twice the base poverty level. Of these, the vast majority were in employment. Respondents were particularly likely to be poor if they were not categorised as disabled or elderly by the benefit system, but still claiming unemployment or short-term sickness benefits, as were those who had a broken employment record. Indeed, this latter group were more likely to be poor than those who had never worked.

The causes of poverty among disabled people

Employment and earnings

Disability results in a loss of earnings when an individual is unable to work. This can happen because the impact of the disability truly makes it impossible to sustain employment. More commonly it happens because of discrimination by employers (Barnes, 1991; Layard *et al.*, 1978; Walker and Walker, 1991). The low incomes of disabled people are sometimes viewed as inevitable. People with impairments are seen as *inevitably* unable to participate in employment. If they do work, it is assumed that their productivity will be lower, which warrants lower earnings.

This is wrong on two counts. First, disabled people are *not* necessarily less productive than their non-disabled colleagues. The evidence is that many are at least as productive as able-bodied colleagues (Lunt and Thornton, 1993). Second, it overlooks the fact that work can be organised to include as well as exclude people with impairments. Oliver (1990) highlights the mechanisation and growing speed of factory work from the industrial revolution onwards as a key to the exclusion of disabled people from contemporary labour markets. Many disabled people need work tasks to be organised flexibly and to be able to work part-time if they are to sustain employment. Prescott-Clarke (1990), in a large survey concerned with disability and employment, found that significant proportions of respondents needed flexibility in either work tasks (28 per cent), or working hours, to be able to sustain employment. Indeed, these were mentioned by more disabled people than adjustments to the physical environment of work. Only 8 per cent of those interviewed mentioned changes to the physical environment. Clearly, employers do not respond to these needs for flexible working.

Finally, to put this issue in context, it is important to remember that 'disability' is a continuum. Very few of us are totally 'able' for all of our working lives. Tapping the employment potential of people with impairments, and their talents, is of enormous importance for the economy.

Manifestly, access to paid employment is a key determinant of the living standards of disabled people, as for other groups in the population. Yet research consistently shows that they are much less likely to be in paid work. Only 31 per cent of disabled people of working age were in paid work in 1985, compared with 69 per cent of the population as a whole (Smyth, 1989). Some 78 per cent of all disabled people live in households where there are no earners. Many of these are retired, but even amongst those of working age, half are in non-earning households (Martin and White, 1988). Although legislation (The Disabled Persons [Employment] Act 1944) requiring employers to employ a minimum of at least 3 per cent registered disabled people was introduced in 1944, this was never effectively enforced. Only ten prosecutions have been brought since 1975, and 80 per cent of employers currently fail to meet the quota requirements (Gooding, 1994). Most provisions of this Act have been repealed by the Disability Discrimination Act 1995; the impact of the new legislation remains to be seen.

Those disabled people who do work earn significantly less than their non-disabled peers (Martin and White, 1988). This is not related to the numbers of hours worked; the vast majority (94 per cent) of disabled men in employment work full-time, while disabled women are no more likely to work part-time than non-disabled women (Martin *et al.*, 1989). However, disabled people are more likely to be working in lower status and less well-paid jobs. Fewer, for example, have professional or managerial posts; only 18 per cent of men compared with 28 per cent of men in the general population (ibid.). (These differences, in both earnings and types of work, are less marked for disabled women, as women generally have lower earnings and lower status jobs than men.) The overwhelming majority of disabled people are thus either not employed or employed in jobs which are poorly paid, undemanding and unrewarding; the type of work which has been characterised as 'underemployment' (Barnes, 1991; Walker, 1982).

The additional costs of disability

We have seen that disability is associated with low income. It also creates special demands on income, which can intensify the poverty of many disabled people. Disabled people frequently incur additional costs because of their condition: a special diet, special equipment or adaptations to their homes, extra heating because they are at home most of the time and feel the cold because they cannot move around easily, and so on. The lack of suitable public services can mean they have to spend more than someone who is able-bodied, for instance when they have to use taxis because public transport is not accessible or to pay for assistance at home which health and social services do not provide. Estimating the level of these additional costs is a complex and, inevitably, a politicised activity. All the methods that have been used are open to criticism (for a useful discussion of the merits of various approaches, see Berthoud, 1993).

Three approaches have been used in research on the costs of disability. First, disabled people have been asked to identify items on which they spend extra and to give an average weekly figure for their extra spending on each item. Hyman (1977) calculated that disabled people were spending £14 a week (or 24 per cent of their incomes) on the additional costs of disability; Buckle (1984) estimated additional weekly costs of £19.50 in 1981; Stowell and Day (1983) found that disabled people were spending an additional £3.36 per week on grocery shopping alone. The OPCS disability surveys suggested average additional costs of £6.10 a week, using this approach. Costs rose with severity of disability. For those in the highest severity category, extra expenditure exceeded £20 per week (Martin and White, 1988). However, the OPCS figures were regarded as excessively conservative by disability organisations. The Disability Income Group undertook two further surveys (Thompson *et al.*, 1988 and Thompson *et al.*, 1990) concerned solely with additional costs. These estimated the average at around £50 per week. A second approach is to compare the actual expenditure of disabled people on various items with that of non-disabled people. This approach was used by Baldwin (1985), who replicated the Family Expenditure Survey for families with disabled children and compared their spending with that of families in the general population. Matthews and Truscott (1990) took a similar approach in a special analysis of the Family Expenditure Survey designed to complement the OPCS surveys. This, again, demonstrated additional expenditure on some items (fuel, consumer durables, tobacco and services) and reduced expenditure on others (clothing and transport).

A third approach seeks to estimate the costs of disability by looking at the consequences of such extra costs for spending on other items, and thus for disabled people's living standards. Basically, this approach aims to establish the level of income disabled people would need in order to achieve lifestyles comparable with those of non-disabled people. Berthoud *et al.* (1993) adopted this approach in their comparison of OPCS and FES data. Their re-analysis of the OPCS data demonstrated not only that deprivation (measured by inability to take part in social activities and absence of consumer durables) was common among disabled people, but also that it was strongly related to low income and to severity of disability. Strikingly, Berthoud *et al.*'s (1993) re-analysis of the OPCS data produced a much higher figure for extra costs than had been produced by the OPCS researchers, with an average estimated at around £30 a week.

The costs of personal assistance

Help required with personal care and a range of social and domestic tasks, referred to variously as 'care' or 'personal assistance' results in additional costs for disabled people. The history of public provision to meet these costs is complex and confused, as, indeed, is the relationship between services providing cash (social security) and care (social services). Some 'care' services are provided free by the NHS, others by social services departments who increasingly charge for them. Until 1988, Supplementary Benefit provided, on an individual and discretionary basis, for the costs disabled people incurred in employing personal and domestic assistance. After the introduction of the simpler Income Support scheme, the costs of personal assistance were provided for in two quite different ways. The severe disability premium was added to the set of premiums which were a central element of the new scheme and meant to reflect the living costs of different claimant groups. The Independent Living Fund (ILF) was also introduced. It was initially aimed at the small group of disabled claimants who needed large amounts of support and who would have lost significantly from the changes. As a charitable trust with a fixed budget replacing a statutory scheme with an open budget, the ILF was initially greeted with considerable scepticism. However, in practice it was warmly received and take-up greatly exceeded expectations. A number of positive evaluations (see, for example, Kestenbaum, 1992; Morris, 1993; Lakey, 1994) have highlighted both the considerable advantages the scheme offers to disabled people – in terms of greater choice and control – and its cost-effectiveness relative to local authority service provision.

Unfortunately, while these positive views were emerging, it was decided to restructure the ILF as part of the 'care in the community' reforms. The ILF closed its doors to new applicants in late 1992. The new version, which started in April 1993, makes local authorities responsible for funding the personal assistance needs up to a cost of £200 per week. Disabled people of working age whose assistance costs are greater than this (but do not exceed £500 per week in total) are now entitled to apply to the Independent Living (1993) Fund. Tight income and capital criteria, combined with the requirement for the local authority to provide the first £200 of funding, have led to low take-up of the 'new' ILF; only 21 per cent of the fund's budget was spent in the first year. (George, 1994). One consequence of these changes has been to increase pressure for local authorities to make direct cash payments to disabled people to enable them to choose and manage the support they want, rather than relying on the judgements of professionals. However, it was illegal, under the terms of the 1948 National Assistance Act, to make such payments. Bowing to pressure for reform, the government introduced draft legislation in 1996 which empowers local authorities to make direct cash payments in lieu of all, or part of, the services a disabled person is assessed as needing (under the NHS and Community Care Act 1990). The impact of this change is potentially considerable. However, it further complicates the relationship between social security and local authority provision for disabled people.

Disability and social security

Income replacement benefits

Social security benefits are a vital source of income for disabled people. The OPCS surveys established that for three-quarters of disabled people in Britain, benefits were their main source of income (Martin and White, 1988). Many were receiving 'mainstream' income-replacement benefits such as Retirement Pension or Income Support. Only a third of disabled people of working age received a benefit aiming *specifically* to provide an income for disabled people, such as Invalidity (now Incapacity) Benefit or Severe Disablement Allowance (Martin and White, 1988; Walker and Walker, 1991). This highlights gaps in social security provision for disabled people which can be traced back to the origins of the British social insurance scheme.

In reviewing the social security system, Beveridge found a patchwork of existing benefits for disability paying very different amounts according to its cause. Those injured in military service or at work received generous benefits as of right. Those whose impairments or illnesses had other causes usually had to rely on means-tested social assistance. He originally proposed a unified scheme of disability benefits which would remove such distinctions, but this was rejected. The scheme which was adopted failed to provide for the 'civilian' disabled – people who did not have a claim to War Pensions or Industrial Injuries benefits. People who were disabled or had a long-term illness had to supplement their flat-rate Sickness Benefit by claiming means-tested social assistance.

Not until 1971 was a specific income-replacement benefit, Invalidity Benefit, introduced for some people in this group. Eligibility for Invalidity Benefit requires a history of participation in employment and of National Insurance contributions. Clearly, however, insurance-based benefits cannot adequately provide for people who are unable to work or have a poor, or interrupted, contributions record because they have been severely disabled at birth or early in life, or suffer from chronic illness. Non-contributory Invalidity Pension (NCIP) was introduced four years after Invalidity Benefit, in 1975, to provide an income for people in this situation. NCIP was regarded as a very partial victory by disabled activists for two reasons. First, it was paid at a significantly lower rate than the contributory Invalidity Pension, to maintain the differential between people who did and did not make National Insurance contributions, and married women were not initially eligible for the new benefit. The reason given for their exclusion was that they 'would have been at home in any case'. Pressure against this manifestly discriminatory stance resulted in the creation, in 1977, of a special benefit for disabled women without a contributions record: Housewives Non-Contributory Pension (HNCIP). Eligibility criteria for this benefit centred on proof of inability to carry out domestic tasks. This was widely regarded as discriminatory and unworkable and, following successful challenges under European Community sex discrimination legislation, both NCIP and HNCIP were replaced by a new benefit – Severe Disablement Allowance (SDA) – in 1984.

The new benefit was more equitable. However, it was also more restrictive in coverage, since eligibility now depended on demonstrating functional disability of 80 per cent. SDA was originally set at a flat rate, well below the level of Invalidity Benefit. Although age-related additions have subsequently been added, its level remains well below that of the contributory benefit and of means-tested benefit levels. In consequence, the great majority of recipients still rely on IS to bring their incomes to the very modest sums provided by IS.

Benefits for extra costs

The 1970s saw acceptance of the need to provide the 'civilian' disabled with help towards the extra costs of disability. This had previously been accepted only in relation to people receiving War Pensions or Industrial Injuries benefits, and to the very small number able to establish liability through the legal system. Two new benefits, Attendance and Mobility Allowance, were introduced, in 1971 and 1975, respectively. Mobility Allowance was intended to meet the extra costs of transport, and the payment of a cash allowance, instead of the notoriously unsafe three-wheeled vehicle previously supplied, was a welcome move to greater consumer choice. What Attendance Allowance was for was less clear-cut. The original policy aim in introducing it was to provide help with disability-related costs of all kinds. However, its name, and the fact that the eligibility criteria relate to care and supervision needs, encouraged the misconception that the purpose of Attendance Allowance was to pay for care costs. As benefits that were relatively generous and tax-free, Mobility and Attendance Allowance have played a major part in improving the living standards of disabled people. However, the fact that their incomes are generally low means that disabled people are often forced to use them on general living costs rather than extra needs arising from disability (Berthoud, 1993).

Recent developments

Disability benefits were not included in the major review of social security benefits in 1985; the rationale for their being excluded was that any review needed to wait for the findings of the OPCS disability surveys, then in the field. When the results of these surveys were published in 1988/9, a major review *was* carried out, but this was largely an internal exercise done without public consultation. The lack of consultation shows clearly in its stated objectives:

i   to improve the structure of benefits for disabled people to make it more attuned to their needs and circumstances;

ii   to promote independence where this is feasible and sensible and in particular to help disabled people who wish to work to do so;

iii to balance the help given by the different benefits so that more is given to those most in need, especially those disabled at birth or early in life;

iv   to avoid duplication with other sources of help.

(DSS, 1990)

Significantly, the simplification of an acknowledged complex and inequitable system was not identified as an objective, although disabled people's organisations had campaigned continuously since the mid-1960s for the replacement of the current patchwork of benefits by a more coherent benefit structure based on the severity of disability rather than its cause. Their goal was, and remains, a comprehensive 'disability income' which encompasses earnings replacement, extra costs and compensation, with benefits levels based on the severity of impairment, not how it had been caused.

The changes that followed from the 1988 review included a restructuring of benefits for extra costs and the introduction of a new work-related benefit and of measures to increase the non-contributory Severe Disablement Allowance for people disabled earlier in life.

Disability Living Allowance

The introduction of Disability Living Allowance (DLA) combines Mobility Allowance and Attendance Allowance into a single benefit. This was a response to findings from the OPCS survey, that while very severely disabled people benefited from Attendance and Mobility Allowances, *moderately* disabled people were often excluded from these benefits, though they also incurred extra costs. The new benefit therefore introduced a lower level of mobility allowance (for people able to walk but needing guidance or supervision to do so). It also introduced a lower level of 'care' allowance (for people who need help with personal care or domestic tasks for around an hour a day). While DLA is now a single benefit, it has a very complex structure, with two components (Mobility and Care) and five different levels of payment. To complicate matters further, the old Attendance Allowance is retained for people over 65.

An evaluation of DLA (Sainsbury *et al.*, 1995) concludes that it has succeeded in reaching some moderately disabled people who failed to qualify under the previous criteria. However, lobbying from pressure groups continues to focus on groups who are still excluded – deaf people who need to pay interpreters, for example. These claims are resisted by the Department of Social Security, concerned that the scope and cost of the new benefit will go significantly beyond the original policy intention. If past history is anything to go by, this pressure for expansion will be difficult to resist. A different kind of concern relates to the decision to align the new benefit more clearly with the costs of care, rather than extra costs in general. Any ambiguity about the purpose of Attendance Allowance has now been removed; DLA (Care) is clearly meant to provide help with the costs of care. This has already had the effect of encouraging local authorities to rule that DLA should be used to pay for community care services. This stance is hotly disputed by disabled people and their organisations, not least since disabled people have to buy many kinds of 'care' other than those provided by social services departments.

Disability Working Allowance

Disability Working Allowance (DWA) was introduced to fill a gap in social security provision for disabled people who want to work but cannot manage a full working week. It provides a supplement to low earnings for disabled people employed sixteen hours or more a week. DWA stops short of being a true partial capacity benefit (the goal of disability campaigners for many years) by including a means test which limits its value. Unlike DLA, which has exceeded expectations of take-up, DWA has not reached its target group. It had been estimated that around 50,000 people would be eligible, but 18 months after its introduction only 4,300 were receiving it. Research on DWA (Rowlingson and Berthoud, 1994) suggests that the main factor influencing its low take-up is a shortage of employment opportunities, rather than ignorance or misunderstanding of the benefit or its likely value.

... Some You Lose? Restricting Invalidity Benefit

This expansion of provision was followed, five years later, by a major restriction in social security protection for people whose working lives are interrupted – or terminated – by illness or disability. The background to this development lies in government concern about the rising cost of social security. Expenditure on invalidity benefits plays a significant part in this. Like other Western countries, the UK has experienced a significant rise in the number of people claiming invalidity benefits in the 1980s and 1990s (Lonsdale and Seddon, 1994). Political discussion of this phenomenon in the UK has focused on the financial incentive to claim invalidity benefits rather than the much lower benefits available to those simply unemployed – and to suggest that people claiming invalidity benefit are not 'genuinely' disabled. This is questionable. Research suggests that most of the increase is caused by people staying on Invalidity Benefit longer, not by a rise in the number of people claiming it in the first place (Berthoud, 1993). This, in turn, reflects demographic change (increasing ill-health in an ageing population) coupled with decreasing labour market opportunities. Nevertheless, Invalidity Benefit was replaced in 1995 by Incapacity Benefit. The new benefit cuts benefit levels and restricts access to benefit in a number of ways. Most importantly, it makes entitlement to benefit after 28 weeks dependent on a test of incapacity for *any* paid work. The new 'test' is based on an assessment which 'scores' a range of functional abilities; people who score below a certain level are deemed capable of paid work. The DSS argues that the new test provides a more objective, and more equitable, measure of (in)capacity for work. This claim is strongly disputed by welfare rights and disability organisations, academics, and some medical practitioners. They reject the notion that capacity for employment can be measured objectively; and assert that functional ability is, in fact, a very poor measure of a person's ability to carry out paid work. It certainly does not capture important factors such as difficulties created by the design of buildings, the organisation of work or discrimination by employers. What is clear is that the new benefit will create major savings for government by excluding large numbers of claimants, current and potential. It is estimated that 220,000 fewer will be eligible, of whom only a minority are likely to succeed in finding paid work. Many of the remainder will have no entitlement to benefits or will have to claim Income Support as simply unemployed, thus falling into deeper poverty (Berthoud, 1993).

The overall impact of these new developments is difficult to assess. In terms of income replacement, the picture is one of advances in some areas balanced by reverses in others. Severe Disablement Allowance and Disability Working Allowance recognise the *principle* that people who are severely disabled, particularly early in life, should have an income that recognises their disability and helps them to build on partial capacity for paid work. In *practice*, however, these benefits are paid at levels which make it difficult to rise much above the level of Income Support and do not create strong incentives to take paid work, should it be offered. For people whose illness or disability occurs later, during their working life, the restrictions imposed by the new Incapacity Benefit may, again, lead to reliance on means-tested benefits. This not only results in low income but also the threat of constant policing to ensure that they are truly incapable of finding paid work. In terms of extra costs benefits, the picture is more straightforwardly one of progress, though disability and welfare rights activists argue that much remains to be done: DLA still excludes some disabled people who have extra costs and the level of benefit for the most severely disabled is inadequate. Above all, no real progress has been made towards the goal disabled activists (and DIG in particular) have been pursuing for thirty years: an adequate, coherent, comprehensive, disability income based on degree, and not cause, of impairment. As this chapter demonstrates, benefits for disability remain a complex maze, and the amount of money people get is still tied to how they became disabled, not their needs.

The impact of disability on household incomes

Disability in one family member will often affect the living standards of others; households containing a disabled person are frequently poor households (Matthews and Truscott, 1990). This is partly caused by the low level of disability benefits. It also reflects the fact that relatives are involved in giving care and support, which reduces the hours they can work or prevents them from working, and the benefits available to them are equally low. If poverty is to be prevented, income maintenance policies must address the needs of both disabled people and those who support them.

The costs of caring

There is considerable research evidence of the financial effects of providing 'informal' care for a disabled person. Baldwin (1985) and Smyth and Robus (1989) have documented the effects of caring for a disabled child on both mothers' and fathers' labour force participation.

The latter study found that a third of families had no earner in the household. Evandrou and Winter's (1993) analysis of General Household Survey data on carers reports that most have to leave the labour market, or substantially reduce their hours of work in order to accommodate their caring responsibilities. Berthoud (1993) found evidence that, while some women became the main earner when their partner became disabled, this was much less common when women were involved in caring activities for more than an hour or so each day. Glendinning (1983) has documented the extra expenses encountered by relatives caring for older or disabled kin.

Invalid Care Allowance (ICA), a non-contributory benefit intended for carers unable to work because of caring commitments, was introduced in 1975. As noted earlier in this chapter, the legacy of Beveridge was evident in assumptions about married women's financial dependence on their husbands, reflected in the initial lack of benefits for married women who were ill or disabled. This story is repeated with ICA. Married women were excluded from ICA until 1986, when a test case (the Drake case) established that the ICA criteria breached European law on the equal treatment of men and women.

ICA has been subject to continuous criticism since its inception (Baldwin and Parker, 1991). The driving force behind this criticism is that it is a benefit which does not adequately reflect carers' situations, or meet their needs. Entitlement depends not only on the carer's situation but that of the person cared for – they have to be receiving AA or the higher or middle rates of DLA (Care). It is paid at a very low rate compared to other earnings replacement benefits (£36.60 a week in 1996 as against £48.25 unemployment benefit). Because of restrictive entitlement conditions, it is estimated to reach only 10 per cent of those potentially eligible (McLaughlin, 1991). It is too low to replace carers' earnings, much less *pay* them for the minimum working week of 35 hours required for eligibility. It does not reflect the extra expenses carers often incur; whether the person cared for is a child (Baldwin, 1985; Glendinning, 1983), a young adult (Hirst, 1985), a partner (Parker, 1992), or an elderly parent (Glendinning, 1990; Levin *et al.*, 1989; Nissel and Bonnerjea, 1982). It stops quickly (after four weeks) when the person cared for dies or goes into residential care, with no period of grace for the carer to re-adjust, recover or retrain.

Marginal changes to ICA have been made in response to these criticisms, the most notable being to the amount carers can earn before sacrificing entitlement completely. In 1996 this stood at £50 a week. The original amount allowed carers to do very little paid work before losing entitlement to ICA. However, a series of calls for fundamental reform of social security provision for carers, including proposals by the House of Commons Social Security Committee has gone unheeded. This is troubling, and also puzzling, in view of the fact that government openly acknowledges family carers as the linch-pin of community care policy and expresses great concern about their continued willingness to go on caring.

Small change?

If the 1980s saw a trend towards increased coverage in benefits for disabled people, this has been balanced by new restrictions and a steady erosion of their living standards. Opportunities for paid work have been seriously constrained by mass unemployment and the continuing failure to enforce 'quota' legislation (Glendinning, 1991). Benefit reforms have reduced the levels of income-replacement benefits, while also tightening eligibility criteria, with damaging effects on independence and autonomy as well as living standards. Disabled people were also badly affected by the 'simplification' of Income Support after 1988. The replacement of individually assessed additions by standard premiums, and the introduction of the discretionary, cash-limited, Social Fund in place of grants for essential items, reduced the level and flexibility of help with the extra costs arising from disability. As Walker and Walker (1991) notes somewhat wryly, many of these cuts were implemented while the OPCS surveys were still collecting data on which policy was to be reviewed.

The introduction of Value Added Tax on domestic fuel has also had a disproportionate impact on disabled people (Gathorne-Hardy, 1994; Hutton and Hardman, 1994). Finally, the widespread move to charge users for social services (including some previously supplied free, by the health service), not only widens the range of means-tests to which disabled people are exposed, but will also deepen the poverty in which most of them live. Most social services authorities take into account benefits such as DLA (Care) and Attendance Allowance, which are excluded from assessment for benefit purposes. Many also impose minimum charges, regardless of how low a service user's income is. Central government's principal grant to local authorities, the Revenue Support Grant, now assumes that they will recover 9 per cent of the cost of providing domiciliary services from charges. This, together with other financial pressures, has created an almost irresistible pressure to increase revenue from charges. Only a handful of authorities still provide free home-care services (Balloch and Robertson, 1995; Baldwin and Lunt, 1996). Most fail to assess accurately whether service users *can* afford to contribute to the cost of their services. A wide range of approaches exists to assessing whether, and how much, users can afford to pay. Virtually all take Income Support levels as a proxy for a minimum income level, despite the large body of evidence that they are not adequate for a reasonable quality of life. In addition, virtually no authority makes allowance for the actual outgoings, and extra costs, of disabled individuals. Many aim to allow for extra costs, but do so at a general level and restrict this to 'special' expenses such as heating, diet and laundry. None consider social or recreational expenditure as relevant (National Consumer Council, 1995). The consequence of these multiple demands on their incomes are lower standards and quality of life, increased problems with debt, and, in some cases, care needs that go unmet (Chetwynd and Ritchie, 1996; Grant, 1995).

Conclusion

Nearly a century after social policy began to address the problem of disability, chronic illness and disability still carry a high risk of long-term poverty, not only for the disabled individual, but for the entire household, particularly where members of the household are involved in providing care and support for the disabled person. Despite the fact that the benefit system recognises the two keys areas of lost earnings and increased costs, the evidence is that it fails to adequately compensate for these problems. There are a number of reasons for this, including an over-reliance on contributory benefits and the low levels of these benefits. The disability benefit system remains fragmented, with too much emphasis on the origin of disability, rather than its effects. The interface between social security and the labour market is also problematic; there is only limited provision for those with partial capacity for work, and the emphasis is on proving the genuine disability of individuals rather than looking at the attitudes of employers. There is thus considerable scope for the improvement of the social security system to create a positive emphasis on rehabilitation, rather than policing individuals. This would be consistent with developing understandings of the social construction of disability, yet social security does not seem to be perceived as a key issue by disabled people at present. There may be a number of reasons for this, including a general air of pessimism about the possibility of benefit reforms in a period of cutbacks, and a concentration on the need for anti-discrimination legislation to ensure access to employment and other areas of social life. The debate has tended to be framed in terms which suggest that social rights and civil rights are mutually exclusive. Burkhauser (1992) has argued that the Americans with Disabilities Act allows employers to 'cream off' an elite of highly educated disabled people who are articulate enough to demand their legal rights. At the same time some disabled activists have argued that equal access to employment would remove the need for benefits. The reality is that both civil rights – to freedom from discrimination in both public and private life – and social rights – to service provision and cash benefits – are necessary weapons if the link between poverty and disability is to be severed.

Postscript

Since the election of the Labour Goverment in May 1997, there have been several interesting, if as yet inconclusive, developments in the policy relating to disabled people. Perhaps most significant has been the inclusion of disabled people as a target group for the New Deal initiative intended to get unemployed people back to work. This has led to the provision of £195 million in funding for pilot projects to improve the employment prospects of disabled people. At the same time, developments in social security policy have caused concern; the so-called Benefit Integrity Project has sought to eliminate large numbers of claims for Incapacity Benefit, and the possibility of means-testing benefits for extra costs has been mooted repeatedly. Promises to extend anti-discrimination legislation also appear to be slow in reaching fruition; cost constraints are being blamed. It is too early to say what effects these current developments will have on the situation of disabled people described in this chapter. What is encouraging is that they have fostered a renewed recognition amongst the disability movement of the importance of both social security benefits and employment in preventing poverty.

Notes

1 Such as arthritis and back pain.
2 Percentages exceed 100 as information collected on all disabling conditions.
3 The incomes of disabled people over pension age were similar to those of non-disabled pensioners. That reflects the lower incomes of all pensioners relative to the general population.

References

Aylward, M. (1995) 'A new more objective medical assessment for capacity for work in the United Kingdom', paper presented at International Research seminar on 'Issues in Social Security' 17–20 June 1995, Sigtuna, Sweden.

Baldwin, S.M. (1985) *The Costs of Caring: Families with Disabled Children*, London: Routledge and Kegan Paul.

Baldwin, S.M. and Lunt, M. (1996) *Charging Ahead: the Development of Local Authority Charging Policies for Community Care*, Community Care into Practice Series, Bristol: Policy Press.

Baldwin, S. M. and Parker, G. M. (1991) 'Support for informal carers: the role of social security', in G. Dalley *Disability and Social Policy*, London: PSI, pp. 163–198.

Baldwin, S.M., Parker, G.M. and Walker, R. (eds) (1988) *Social Security and Community Care*, Aldershot: Avebury Gower.

Balloch, S. and Robertson, G. (1995) *Charging for Social Care*, London: National Institute for Social Work.

Barnes, C. (1991) *Disabled People in Great Britain and Discrimination*, London: Hurst.

Berthoud, R. (1993) *Incapacity Benefit: Where Will the Savings Come From?*, London: PSI.

Berthoud, R., Lakey, J. and McKay, S. (1993) *The Economic Problems of Disabled People*, London: PSI.

Buckle, J. (1984) *Mental Handicap Costs More*, London: Disablement Income Group.

Burkhauser, R. (1992) 'Beyond stereotypes: public policy and the doubly disabled', *American Enterprise* 3, part 5: 60–69.

Chetwynd, M. and Ritchie, J. (1996) *The Cost of Care*, Bristol: Policy Press.

Crow, L. (1992) 'Reviewing the social model of disability', *Coalition* July, pp. 5–9.

Dalley, G. (1991) *Disability and Social Policy*, London: PSI.

Department of Social Security (1990) *The Way Ahead: Benefits for Disabled People*, London: HMSO.

Doyle, B. (1995) *Disability Discrimination: The New Law*, Jordans.

Evandrou, M. and Winter, D. (1993) *Informal Carers and the Labour Market in Britain*, STICERD WSP/89, London: LSE.

French, S. (1993) 'Disability, impairment or something in between?', in J. Swain, V. Finkelstein, S. French and M. Oliver (eds) *Disabling Barriers, Enabling Environments*, London: Sage and Open University Press.

Gathorne-Hardy, F. (1994) *A Tax on Disability*, London: DIG.

George, M. (1994) 'Paying direct', *Community Care* 25–31 August.

Glendinning, C. (1983) *Unshared Care: Parents and their Disabled Children*, London: Routledge and Kegan Paul.

Glendinning, C. (1990) 'Dependency or interdependency: the incomes of informal carers and the impact of social security', *Journal of Social Policy*, 19 (4): 467–497.

Glendinning, C. (1991) 'Losing ground: social policy and disabled people in Great Britain 1980–90', *Disability Handicap and Society* 6 (1): 3–19.

Gooding, C. (1994) *Disabling Laws, Enabling Acts*, London: Pluto.

Grant, L. (1995) *Disability and Debt: The Experience of Disabled People in Debt*, Sheffield: Sheffield Citizens' Advice Bureau Support Unit.

Hirst, M.A. (1985) 'Social security and insecurity: young people with disabilities in the United Kingdom', *International Social Security Review*, 38 (3): 258–272.

Hutton, S. and Hardman, G. (1994) 'Estimating the effect of VAT on the fuel expenditure of low income households', *Childright* 105: 11–16.

Hyman, M. (1977) *The Extra Costs of Disabled Living*, London: National Fund for Research into Crippling Diseases.

Kestenbaum, A. (1992) *Cash for Care*, London: Independent Living Fund.

Kohli, M., Rein, M. *et al.* (1991) *Time for Retirement*, Cambridge: Cambridge University Press.

Laczko, F. and Phillipson, C. (1991) 'Great Britain: the contradictions of early exit', in M. Kohli, M. Rein *et al. Time for Retirement*, Cambridge: Cambridge University Press.

Lakey, J. (1994) *Caring About Independence: Disabled People and the Independent Living Fund*, London: Policy Studies Institute.

Layard, R., Piachaud, D. and Stewart, M. (1978) *The Causes of Poverty: Background Paper No 5, Royal Commission on Income and Wealth*, London: HMSO.

Levin, E., Sinclair, I., Gorbach, P. with Essame, L. (1989) *Family, Services and Confusion in Old Age*, Aldershot: Avebury.

Lunt, N. and Thornton, P. (1993) *Employment Policies for Disabled People: A Review of Legislation and Services in Fifteen Countries*, Research Report No. 16, London: Department of Employment.

McLaughlin, E. (1991) *Social Security and Community Care: the Case of Invalid Care Allowance*, London: HMSO.

Martin, J. and White, A. (1988) *The Financial Circumstances of Disabled Adults Living in Private Households*, London: HMSO.

Martin, J., Meltzer, H. and Elliot, D. (1988) *The Prevalence of Disability Among Adults*, London: HMSO

Martin, J., White, A. and Meltzer, H. (1989) *Disabled Adults: Services, Transport and Employment*, London: HMSO.

Matthews, A. and Truscott, P. (1990) *Disability, Household Income and Expenditure: A Follow-up Survey of Disabled Adults in the Family Expenditure Survey*, London: HMSO.

Morris, J. (1992) *Personal and Political: A Feminist Perspective on Researching Disability*,

Morris, J. (1993) *Community Care or Independent Living?*, York: Joseph Rowntree Foundation.

National Consumer Council (1995) *Charging Consumers for Social Services*, London: NCC.

Nissel, M. and Bonnerjea, L. (1982) *Family Care of the Handicapped Elderly*, London: Policy Studies Institute.

Oliver, M. (1990) *The Politics of Disablement*, Basingstoke: Macmillan.

Parker, G.M. (1992) *With this Body: Caring and Disability in Marriage*, Buckingham: Open University Press.

Prescott-Clarke, P. (1990) *Employment and Handicap*, London: SCPR.

Rowlingson, K. and Berthoud, R. (1994) *Evaluating the Disability Working Allowance*, London: PSI.

Sainsbury, R., Hirst, M. and Lawton, D. (1995) *An Evaluation of Disability Living Allowance and Attendance Allowance*, London: HMSO.

Smyth, M. and Robus, N. (1989) *The Financial Circumstances of Families with Disabled Children Living in Private Households*, London: HMSO.

Stowell, R. and Day, F. (1983) *Tell Me What You Want and I'll Get It For You*, London: DIG.

Thompson, P., Buckle, J. and Curtice, J. (1990) *Short Changed by Disability*, London: DIG.

Thompson, P., Buckle, J. and Lavery, M. (1988) *Not the OPCS Survey: Being Disabled Costs More Than They Said*, London: DIG.

UPIAS (1976) *Fundamental Principles of Disability*, London: Union of Physically Impaired Against Segregation.

Wadensjo, E. (1991) 'Sweden – partial exit', in M. Kohli, M. Rein *et al. Time for Retirement*, Cambridge: Cambridge University Press.

Walker, A. (1982) *Underqualified and Underemployed*, Basingstoke: Macmillan.

Walker, A. and Walker, L. (1991) 'Disability and financial need: the failure of the social security system', in G. Dalley *Disability and Social Policy*, London: PSI.

Wood, P. (1981) *International Classification of Impairments, Disabilities and Handicaps*, Geneva: WHO.

Wright, F. (1986) *Left to Care Alone*, Aldershot: Gower.

Zarb, G. (ed.) (1995) *Removing Disabling Barriers*, London: PSI.

8 Social security and poverty

Women's business

Eithne McLaughlin

Women are, and always have been, the main users of social security provision, although most social security systems and sub-systems have been created with men in mind as the primary claimants. Women are also the majority of the poor whether measured on the basis of household or individual incomes and assets. In order to evaluate the extent to which social security provision has alleviated or prevented poverty, it is therefore essential to examine how and why women's greater use of social security has not prevented higher levels of poverty among women than men. Such a gender analysis involves examining the origins and development of social security systems, in order to see what assumptions, if any, were made about the roles and positions of women and men in society and economy by policy architects. It also involves analysis of the roles and positions held by women and men socially and economically, and comparison with the assumptions about these underlying the system of provision.

In the UK, women form the majority of recipients of all the major benefits apart from Unemployment Benefit (now Jobseekers Allowance), Invalidity Benefit (now Incapacity Benefit) and Industrial Injury Benefit (Lister, 1992). This is not a new situation – from the days of the Poor Law to the present, women have been the majority of those 'dependent' on welfare. While men dominate the work-related National Insurance benefits, women dominate the lesser system of means-tested benefits and non-contributory benefits, entitlement to most of which derive in some way from their relationships with others. It has been as mothers, including lone mothers, and the majority of older and disabled people, and those providing unpaid assistance to them, that women have claimed social security benefits. In 1993, for instance, about 7 million women received Child Benefit, about 9.2 million, Income Support (of whom 6.5 million were over pension age), and about 0.5 million, Family Credit (Millar, 1995, p. 53), to mention just a few. Yet more women are not visible in their own right as benefit recipients – almost 1 million were living on Income Support claimed by their partners in 1992 (ibid.) while Esam and Berthoud (1991) estimated that about 3.7 million husbands received some kind of social security benefit in respect of their wives.

Although the social security system has failed to end poverty among either women or men, it has nevertheless been extremely important in reducing the income inequalities between men and women which result from their different labour market incomes and in providing women with some alternative (albeit a 'poor' alternative) to traditional marriage. This is not to say that the social security system is without its inadequacies in relation to women, but rather that it has been 'Janus-faced' in terms of the development of gender relations and the reduction of gender inequalities. In critique of the social security system, two main topics emerge as important, on the one hand, why it should be that women's positions as wives and mothers should result in their reliance on the least advantageous parts of the social security system and, on the other, why it should be that women's paid work does not bring them into the net of the main National Insurance benefits to the same extent that men's paid work does. In terms of substantive areas of research, the most recent analyses have focused on the interconnection of these two topics through, first, analyses of the impact of means-tested in-work benefits on wives' and mothers' labour supply and, second, the meaning and impact of the Child Support Act. In this chapter little attention will be paid to pensions issues, despite their topicality, because these are covered in Chapter 5 of this volume. Theoretically, the most recent focus in this field has been international comparisons of the 'two-track' gendered nature of many Western social security systems, and relatedly the extent to which social security systems assume adult women to be financially dependent upon male partners rather than financially independent.

Women, social security and the regulation of marriage

Approaches to, or schools of thought about, social security have differed mainly in terms of the degree to which they have focused on one of the three main purposes or 'functions' of social security. These are: to prevent or alleviate poverty; to regulate or provide discipline for the labour market; to regulate lifestyles and especially 'family' forms, in favour of the married state. Thus the Fabian tradition has framed its critique in terms of how well the social security system has prevented or alleviated poverty; and the degree to which the social security has succeeded in making the income distribution more egalitarian than it would otherwise be (if left to the market alone). Meanwhile, those on the more radical left, such as Novak (1988), have argued that, under capitalism, social security exists to serve the needs of the labour market, so that the relief of poverty has been a less important objective than the maintenance of work incentives and labour discipline. Similarly, post-structuralist writers, such as Squires (1990), influenced by Foucault, focus on the disciplinary role of social security in relation to paid work (Deacon, 1995, p. 73). Such writers have usefully shown the ways in which the disciplinary nature of social security may be in contradiction with the objective of preventing or alleviating poverty (and especially an objective of substantial degrees of income redistribution); but they have generally omitted analysis of the way social security relies upon specific family forms and relatedly 'recognises' (and hence polices) only some forms of employment and the labour supply of some social groups. It has fallen instead to radical feminist and feminist-socialist writers (such as Land, Lewis, Lister, Millar and Pascall) to develop a critique framed around the relationship between the social security system and 'family' forms. Their critiques have made visible the gender assumptions upon which the social security is based: first, that the appropriate 'unit of intervention' for the state is the household not the individual, and that it is proper for women to derive their 'social security' from the men with whom they live, and, second, that social insecurity results from interruptions to male employment, or failure of the male family wage. Through this, they have developed a critique of the concept of poverty itself.

These assumptions have a long history – throughout the history of the Poor Law, women were a majority of adult recipients of relief but it was assumed that if the problem of male unemployment were solved, then women's need for relief would disappear. This assumption was, of course, totally incompatible with the reality of eighteenth- and nineteenth-century working-class life, which involved recurrent unemployment for both sexes, early and sudden death of men, and significant levels of conception and motherhood outside marriage. Such assumptions continued, however, into the National Insurance Act of 1911 and, of course, the Beveridge Report of 1942. Beveridge treated single women (that is, never married women) as 'honorary' men – in other words, if they abandoned their simulated maleness by having children while unmarried, or by caring for elderly parents rather than working in the labour market, then they had to forsake their preferable position compared with married women. As regards married women, Beveridge made clear that their financial security should be derived from their husbands because 'during marriage most women will not be gainfully occupied … The attitude of the housewife to gainful employment outside the home is not and should not be the same as the single woman – she has other duties' (Beveridge, 1942, pp. 50–51).

Whatever the inadequacies of this approach in terms of addressing poverty amongst married women, it is important to recognise the limitations inherent in this approach because of its role in relation to 'policing' adults' emotional and sexual lives. This has been clear in two main ways: first, the problem of what to do with women whose marriages end and, second, what to do about women having heterosexual relationships outside marriage. Beveridge himself recognised the insecurities for women inherent in his reliance on marriage as the source of women's social security and proposed an analogy between marriage/housewifery and paid work (Lister, 1994). The end of marriage would be like the end of employment so there should be widows' benefits and separation/divorce benefits. Beveridge's proposals for the latter were not accepted after the War nor since. Marriage breakdown presents a dilemma which is not easily solved in an insurance system. It is undeniably a 'risk' to the housewife whose financial security in both the short term and the long term depends on a husband. But crucial to the insurance notion is that people should not provoke their own need for compensation. Thus notions of guilty and innocent parties in marital breakdown would have to be dispensed with if insurance for divorced and separated women were to be made available. This proved too much for a male-dominated and middle-class political system to bear, partly because it was feared it would make leaving marriage too attractive for women and would reward bad wives. Here, then, was a major loophole – women's social security would depend crucially on marriage but not all women would marry and not all marriages would last. Separated and divorced women were to remain a 'problem' to be picked up in the means-tested safety net, and more recently through the Child Support Act and Agency.

As regards women's heterosexual relationships outside of marriage, if married women's financial security was to be the responsibility of their husbands rather than the state, inevitably the social security system had to be used to determine whether unmarried women, especially unmarried women with children, were really 'single' or simply avoiding dependency on a man (written into marriage) by cohabiting. The principle that heterosexual relationships outside marriage should be treated as if they were the same as marital relationships (that is, that the principle of women's financial dependence on their husbands should be extended to women's male sexual partners) has been present only in the social security system – not in the taxation system. This was because the taxation system bestowed privileges on married couples (actually married men, through the married man's tax allowance) while the social security system did the opposite (two 'single' people's benefits being larger than a couple's). To the extent that both the taxation and the social security systems were devoted to discipling adult sexual relations and promoting marriage, then the treatment of cohabiting couples as 'the same as' married couples in social security but not in taxation made sense (Fairbairns, 1985).

During the 1970s this 'cohabitation rule' came under considerable attention because of the way it 'sexualised' the administration of social security. Women who had male lodgers, women who had a male friend who visited a lot, and women whose ex-partners maintained access to their children, were all likely to be suspected of cohabitation. Enforcement of the cohabitation rule meant investigation of women's personal and sexual lives, direct and surreptitious, formal investigation and informal spying by social security staff and neighbours. This 'sexualisation' of the administration of social security has more recently taken on a new form through the operation of the Child Support Act and Agency, discussed below.

In addition, the attribution of married women's financial security to their husbands, rather than the social security system, has meant that the social security system has relied on husbands to 'claim for' their wives and then to distribute the resultant income in whatever way they saw fit. The 1985 Green and White Papers on social security reform, for example, stated that the social security system had to 'trust' men as breadwinners to distribute their income (either benefits or earnings) 'responsibly'. It is worth noting the use of the word 'responsibly' here, in preference to, say, 'equitably'. This signifies the way the state, through the social security system, has not only relied on a particular family form (in design and administrative terms) but has also approved a specific kind of familial relationship – that it is a man's decision how much money his wife (or cohabitee) and children 'need'. Thus the welfare of married women and children has been deemed to be the responsibility of individual men not the state. This point is taken up further in the next section to relation to its implications for women's experience of poverty.

Women, social security and poverty

As Deacon (1995, p. 76) states, Beveridge's insurance scheme was ill suited to a world in which growing proportions (now a majority) of mothers with dependent children were in full-time or part-time work, in which growing proportions of marriages (now one in three) end in divorce or separation, and in which growing proportions (now nearly one-fifth) of families with children were headed by a lone parent. But these were not the only reasons why the post-war system of social security could not possibly fulfil an objective of eradicating poverty. While this is partly to do with the insecurity of marriage over time referred to by Deacon, it is also to do with the insecurity of marriage as a source of income while women are married, and the failure of the social security system to incorporate married women's employment into the National Insurance system, an issue to which we will return below.

As regards marriage as a source of income while the marriage is intact, the idea that the standard of living of all members of a family can be judged by the income of the wage earner or earners was the implicit assumption behind relief of poverty schemes in both the nineteenth and twentieth centuries and indeed (though to a lesser extent) earlier, but it was elevated to an explicit policy principle by Beveridge. In designing the post-war social security system, Beveridge drew heavily, particularly in terms of trying to establish what would be adequate levels of benefits, on the work of Rowntree. While heavily influenced by Rowntree, Beveridge chose not to consider all of the implications of Rowntree's concept of secondary as well as primary poverty. In Rowntree's approach, primary poverty was caused by a household income which was inadequate to cover the basic needs of a family. Secondary poverty, however, was the result of one of two 'failures': either the failure of the wife to manage the household income wisely; or the failure of the husband to distribute what was otherwise an adequate income in such a way as to meet the basic needs of the wife and children. Hence women and children could be malnourished while the 'breadwinner' was not. This was not addressed by Beveridge nor by policy-makers and politicians since, nor even by academics, despite the 'rediscovery of poverty' in the 1950s and 1960s.

Again, it fell to feminist writers in the 1970s and the 1980s (for example, Glendinning and Millar, 1987, 1992; Land, 1983; Pahl 1980, 1989) to 'rediscover' such issues. This is not surprising given that the definition of poverty adopted depends to some extent on what those concerned intend, or expect, to do about it (Alcock, 1993). Non-feminist approaches, whether among academics or policy-makers, necessarily fail to 'see' 'hidden' poverty, since doing something about it would involve policies addressing the nature of relationships between men and women within marriage as well as outside of it. Feminist approaches, however, have repeatedly highlighted, through studies of money management and income sharing within couples, such as Vogler and Pahl (1993), that it is not correct to assume that all the money coming into a household is available in the same way to all family members. Only about one in every five couples have the sort of joint pool that is assumed in the concept of 'family income' which underpins official statistics of 'poverty', or 'below half average income' in 1990s' parlance. In addition, these studies show that the source of income ('his' or 'hers') is important in determining how money is perceived and spent (Millar, 1995, p. 55). Studies of divorced and separated women have also highlighted 'hidden poverty' because they generally show around a third of such women regarding themselves as 'better off' outside than inside marriage (Land, 1994). Given that divorce and separation for women are almost always accompanied by a fall in household income, what such women are describing is the ending of hidden poverty. Such studies also go further and highlight the importance of the experience of autonomy as an element of 'poverty' – that is, 'poverty' is not necessarily only about material outcomes but also about how those outcomes are arrived at. Thus one of the good things about lone motherhood is independence from male financial control (Bradshaw and Millar, 1991; Graham, 1987). The feminist perspective has challenged the definition of poverty as being solely about material conditions and has instead brought attention to the way that poverty is as much about control (of resources and hence important life decisions). Further, the feminist perspective has challenged the notion of dependency put forward by the 'dependency theorists' (Deacon, 1995, p. 73), pointing out that they regard reliance upon a man as normal but reliance upon the state as a problem (see for example, Glendinning and Millar, 1987, 1992; Land, 1983 and Williams, 1989).

This feminist approach to the definition of poverty has led to a number of studies examining sex differences in personal incomes. Davies and Joshi (1994), for example, have estimated that if only minimal 'sharing' of income (specifically sharing of housing costs but nothing else) between couples is assumed, then about 52 per cent of married women were in poverty in 1986 compared with 11 per cent of married men. Evason (1991) used a different approach to make the same point in relation to women in Northern Ireland. Non-employed married women, employed but low-paid women (married or not), and non-employed single women in receipt of benefits – that is, women without access in their own right to income above the level of means-tested benefits – accounted for 75 per cent of adult women in Northern Ireland (Evason, 1991, p. 66). As regards Britain, Esam and Berthoud (1991) calculated that 4.6 million women in 1991–92 had independent incomes of less than £25 a week compared with only 0.4 million men.

Thus although women are more likely than men to receive social security benefit income, this has not resulted in an 'equalisation' of income between the sexes nor has it ended the greater exposure of women than men to poverty, defined in a feminist sense. As Table 8.1 shows, taking all adults in Britain in 1991, women received the equivalent of £23.40 a week per head from social security compared with £19.60 for men. The difference in favour of women – £3.80 – did little to redress the overall income gap between men and women of £99.60 a week. As Table 8.1 shows, the bulk of the income gap – about 70 per cent – was due to differences in earnings, and the other 30 per cent to differences in other forms of income, principally that from self-employment and pensions.

Table 8.1, of course, provides only a crude estimate of the extent to which the social security system 'makes up for' differences in market incomes between men and women, since it takes all ages of adult men and women at a single point in time. A more sophisticated approach, in terms of evaluating the impact of a social security system, or a welfare system generally, is to control for the historical effects of, on the one hand, market change over time and, on the other, welfare change over time, by analysing the effect of the welfare system on a single age cohort over their whole lifecourse, though this inevitably means that assumptions of a stable future have to be made and that the results are not generalisable to the total population. This is the kind of approach taken by a team within the Welfare State Programme at the STICERD, London School of Economics, who have analysed the effects of the welfare system on lifetime incomes and standards of living for a

Table 8.1   Average weekly independent income, 1991, by source and gender, United Kingdom

Income Source	Men	Women	Difference	Women's incomes as % of men's
Earnings	120.80	53.40	−67.40	44.2
Self-employment	28.60	3.80	−24.80	13.3
Social Security	19.60	23.40	+3.80	119.4
Investments	14.60	11.00	−3.60	75.3
Pensions/annuities	14.20	4.90	−9.30	34.5
Other	1.60	3.40	+1.80	212.5
Total	199.50	99.90	−99.60	50.1

Source: Equal Opportunities Commission.

hypothetical cohort of men and women born in 1985, using a microsimulation model called LIFEMOD (Falkingham and Hills, 1995). As they point out, the British welfare state achieves both inter- and intra-personal redistribution, but with the latter being on a larger scale. As it was structured in 1985, between two-thirds and three-quarters of gross lifetime benefits were effectively self-financed, that is, intra-personal redistribution (Evandrou and Falkingham, 1995, p. 182). Nevertheless, the remainder involved inter-personal distribution of a significant level. The lifetime poor are generally the net gainers from the inter-personal redistribution which does occur and the lifetime rich, the net losers. Further, women are overwhelmingly net gainers from the system and men, net losers (ibid., p. 147). Evandrou and Falkingham conclude that men's lifetime original income is almost twice that of women's, that the tax and social security system as it operated in 1985 made a substantial contribution to reducing inequality between men and women, involving a net average lifetime transfer from men to women of between £40,000 and £50,000 (ibid., p. 144), and reducing the ratio of men's and women's net incomes to 1.4 (ibid., p. 182). They point out that whatever private intra-family sharing goes on then acts to further reduce this gender inequality, though as we have noted earlier in this section, such sharing may be problematic for women in so far it remains largely at the discretion of individual men. Importantly, Evandrou and Falkingham also point out that changes to tax and social security between 1985 and 1991 have acted to reduce the scale of redistribution generally, and particularly that between men and women. The changes have meant that the average net lifetime transfer between men and women has fallen by about 20 per cent (or between £8,000 and 10,000 at 1985 prices) (ibid., p. 147).

More generally, Evandrou and Falkingham note that the route to a high lifetime standard of living is different for men and women – for men the labour market is of prime importance whereas for women it remains the marriage market (ibid., p. 182). This is, of course, consistent with the general direction of social security and welfare policy generally in post-war Britain, which has acted to reinforce and sustain the economic importance of marriage for women. The next two sections of this chapter explore this in relation to two main areas of social security policy – the treatment of women's paid work and the treatment of women as mothers, especially lone mothers.

Social security, women's paid work and the family wage

Although Beveridge was primarily concerned with compensating men for unemployment (as well, of course, as other contingencies such as illness and old age), it is also true that 'full employment' for men (the classic '40 hours a week for 40 years'), was assumed – that is, that adult men under 65 should be employed and had no right to support if they choose not to be employed. As a result, there has always been a tension in social security policy between supporting men when they are unemployed and not supporting them so much, or so readily, that they might choose not to be employed (McLaughlin *et al.*, 1989). This is a tension which has become more explicit under the Conservative administration since 1979 and the role of the social security system as an enforcement mechanism of labour market discipline has been the dominant way of analysing the history of the social security system under post-1979 Conservative administrations, a practice which continues. However, analysis of social security in terms of enforcing low-paid work, labour market discipline, and so forth, has focused on the impact upon men and men's employment and unemployment, even though the participation rates of women and men have been converging rapidly over the last two decades. In this section, attention is drawn to some of the ways in which the social security system deals with specific kinds of women's employment, and specific groups of women.

In contrast with disciplining men into paid work, much of the social security system dissuades women from seeing themselves as important labour market workers. For example, fewer unemployed women than men have received unemployment benefit. Many more women than men fail to meet the contribution conditions for unemployment benefit (and, of course, other insurance benefits) (McLaughlin *et al.*, 1999) mostly because of their higher presence in temporary and casual work, intermittent work patterns as a result of breaks to provide care for others, and their higher presence in part-time work, especially part-time work with earnings lower than the threshold at which National Insurance contributions become payable. An estimated 2.25 million working women in the early 1990s were in this latter position (Lister, 1992; McCay *et al.*, 1999).

On the one hand, the failure of so many women to qualify for unemployment benefits results in an underestimation of unemployment (especially long-term unemployment) among women when 'headline' (that is, claimant count) unemployment is discussed. The 1993–94 Labour Force Survey measurement of women reporting that they would like and were seeking a job was two-and-a-half times as great as the claimant count of 'unemployed' women at the time (Callender, 1995, p. 38). An estimated one in four women who lose their jobs do not appear in the claimant count (ibid.). And on the other hand, failure to receive benefit by virtue of one's unemployment (that is, unemployment benefit or income support as an unemployed person) may make individual women less likely to identify, or 'label', themselves as unemployed, even when they have lost a job, are available for and are seeking work. In this sense the social security system contributes to the 'hiding' of, or refusal to grant legitimacy to, certain kinds of barriers to employment (Metcalf, 1992). In addition, the general tightening-up of availability-for-work rules and tests throughout the 1980s and 1990s have made it even more difficult for women with caring responsibilities to establish that they are available for work (for example, claimants may not restrict themselves to being available for part-time work only and must have substitute care arrangements available and capable of being activated within 24 hours).

A further problem (which will be increased by the replacement of 12-months' unemployment benefit with 6-months' Jobseekers Allowance) is that unemployed women who have had no, or have exhausted their, entitlement to unemployment benefit, are unlikely to qualify for benefit unless they are single or have an unemployed partner. In the latter case, it was not until 1983 that women in jobless couples could claim benefit – until then, income support for jobless couples was likely to be claimed by the man in the couple. This has changed as a result of the implementation of the 1979 European Community Directive on Equal Treatment in Social Security, though initially the UK government attempted to limit the impact this change might have by insisting that the claim must be made by the person in the couple who had the most recent labour market contact. This illustrates the general approach taken by the UK government to the Equal Treatment Directive – minimalist reform to remove the most obvious instances of direct discrimination against women in the social security system. Important as this Directive has been in the history of UK social security policy (Lister, 1992), the UK has nevertheless been slow to redress indirect discrimination against women (Millar, 1995; Pascall, 1986). To do so, would have required major reform of the National Insurance contribution (and corresponding benefit entitlement) system. In addition, the EC Directive did not apply to statutory survivors' benefits and pensions. Together, these mean that the contributions of even women earning more than the National Insurance threshold do not carry the same weight as men's – women's contributions will not earn for their partners the right to widow(er)s benefits or retirement pensions. In addition, women are more likely than men to pay 'wasted' contributions. The social security system thus continues to forbid or preclude male financial dependence on women while providing for female dependence on men.

The male breadwinner model in the social security system is also manifest in the impact it has in relation to the incentives, or rather disincentives, poor women have towards participation in employment. While much has been written about social security and incentives for men, very little attention has been paid to women's incentives, though during the 1980s, the increasing political attention paid to lone mothers did feed through into a number of studies of lone mothers' incentives (see for example, McKay and Marsh, 1994 and Bradshaw and Millar, 1991), some of which will be discussed in the next section. Here the focus will be on married and cohabiting women for whom the social security system fairly directly discourages paid work in favour of no work at all in at least two instances – receipt of Family Credit (FC) and the operation of earnings disregards in income support. Family Credit is unambiguously a benefit designed to encourage men into low paid work as the single breadwinner (McLaughlin, 1994a, 1994b); and in practice it is likely that receipt of FC by the man in a couple creates disincentives for their partners to take up paid work in a considerable proportion of families (Marsh and McKay, 1993). If both the man and woman of a couple were in low paid work, it is unlikely the family would qualify for FC (unless both were in part-time jobs, and part-time work among fathers with dependent children remains very unusual indeed). And the marginal deduction rate for women in such FC-recipient families varies between 80 and 95 per cent (taking into account the impact of earnings on housing benefit and community charge as well as Family Credit) (McLaughlin, 1994a, pp. 40–41). Disincentive effects will continue to be present within the Working Families Tax Credit due to replace Family Credit in October 1999, though the effect will be lessened by the availability of a childcare tax credit within WFTC (see McLaughlin *et al.*, 1999).

Family Credit is concerned with putting 'family men' into low-paid work by enabling them to maintain a dependent wife as well as children. This is highly significant from the perspective of preventing poverty – the best way of alleviating and preventing poverty (primary and secondary) among families (that is, men, women and children) is for both partners to earn. Family Credit may appear generous but in fact the resultant overall income level of a household receiving it will remain very substantially below average. In comparison, and notwithstanding women's low pay in employment, even unskilled manual couples with two full-time earners are able to approach average income levels, while others may do so with one full-time and one part-time earner. The adherence in policy to the male family wage/male breadwinner model, despite its inadequacy in relation to the prevention of poverty, is reflected in other parts of the welfare regime as well as in social security. As Millar (1995, p. 58) points out, the government's rationale for the abolition of the Wages Councils in 1994, and hence minimum wages in key industries for women, was that women did not need minimum wage protection because most women live with a partner who is the primary earner. The only Wages Council which was retained was that for the low-pay industry which was most prominently 'male' – agriculture.

Disincentives for women to take paid employment also feature in the way in which the social security system deals with part-time work – the dominant form of work for married women with children. As noted earlier, loss of part-time work is unlikely to be compensated for via social security; while if a woman's partner becomes unemployed, or if she wishes to take up part-time work while her partner is unemployed, all of her earnings above £5 a week will be deducted from the benefit the family would otherwise have received. While the disincentive effects of the low level of these earnings disregards is not the sole explanation for why so few women with unemployed partners engage in part-time work, it does appear to be a significant factor (see McLaughlin, 1994a for a more detailed discussion). Certainly, neither men nor women on income support are given incentives to take part-time work when they are unemployed, even though this is the fastest growing form of work.

'Atypical' (part-time, casual, temporary, seasonal) forms of employment now account for at least a third, and probably fast approaching half, of all jobs (McLaughlin, 1994b), reflecting the UK government's commitment to deregulation of the labour market and enhanced 'flexibility' in the interests of 'competitiveness' (McLaughlin, 1992). Women's contribution to the economy through their take-up of these atypical forms of work (as well as their take-up of full-time work) has been enormous, yet the social security system has failed to recognise and reward this through access to social security protection when such work has been lost, or through encouraging the take-up of this kind of work among poor women in jobless couples.

Social security, care and family forms

Support for families with children

Beveridge's idealisation of housework and childcare – married women's 'vital duties' – might have been assumed to mean that some provision to compensate women for the reduction in labour market opportunities which these duties usually entailed would be included in the post-war social security system. However, Beveridge's assumption that marriage was a partnership in which individual men recognised the vital nature of the work performed by their wives and 'rewarded' them accordingly, meant that he saw no need to introduce compensatory 'care benefits'. Indeed, the only concession to the care provided within families was recognition of the extra costs experienced by families with children, though this was perceived as costs shared by the man and woman and introduced as Family Allowance. Thus, although Eleanor Rathbone in *The Disinherited Family* in 1924 set the case for family allowances firmly in the context of the unpaid nature of housework and childcare, it was economic and demographic rather than feminist arguments which won the day for family allowances and Rathbone and other feminists (such as the Co-operative Women's Guild, see Land and Rose, 1985) in 1945 had to work hard to get the money paid direct to women rather than to men.

Family allowance for second and subsequent children, together with child tax allowances (which benefited men rather than women in terms of net independent income), meant a total package of support in 1946 for a family with three children equivalent to 27 per cent of average male manual earnings (Deacon, 1995, p. 80). Although this was small relative to the contribution a woman's full-time earnings would have made to family income, it was considerably better than the support provided for families with children in more recent times. Neither family allowances nor tax allowances were increased in line with the rise in earnings and prices, and the two were combined in 1977 as Child Benefit. By the late 1970s, support to a family with three children had declined to only 11 per cent of average male manual earnings, although it did recover slightly to 13 per cent in the early 1980s (Deacon and Bradshaw, 1986).

The gradual waning away of support for families with children was probably the result of a number of factors: first, both Labour and Conservative Chancellors of the Exchequer found it easier to increase tax revenues by failing to raise allowances than by the more open method of increasing the actual rates of tax (Deacon, 1995, p. 80); second, the electoral importance of support for families with children waned as the post-war population aged. As Deacon (ibid.) points out, less than one third of voters have dependent children; third, the post-war emphasis on 'building a new nation' (that is, replacement of those lost in War) and the concomitant policy desire to stimulate fertility and home-building (maternalism) also waned as time went on; fourth, the non-means-tested, non-contributory universal nature of Child Benefit was deeply against the grain of modern Conservative ideology.

Whatever the causes, families with children are now disproportionately likely to be in poverty compared with other groups in the population. Nearly two-thirds of those living on incomes that were less than half the national average in 1990–91 were families with children, and 4 million children lived in poor households in 1990–91 compared with 1.4 million in 1979 (Millar, 1993).

Non-contributory benefits

The assumption that women would be at home caring for other people and that women could safely derive their social security from individual men came under increasing attack during the 1970s and the conjunction of the growing disability and women's movement led to the introduction of a number of benefits targeted at people who could not access benefits under the National Insurance system. The strength of campaigning groups was not sufficient, however, to gain entrance to the insurance system for all those outside of it. Instead, a number of 'special category' benefits were introduced – the so-called non-contributory benefits of Invalid Care Allowance (ICA), Non-contributory Invalidity Pension (NCIP) and Housewife's Non-contributory Invalidity Pension (HNCIP). The latter two were targeted at disabled people who had, in the first case, been unable to build an insurance record because of their disability, and in the second case, had been unable to build up an insurance record because of family responsibilities, and were intended to be the equivalent of the contributory Invalidity Benefit. Both the HNCIP and the ICA were directly discriminatory against married women. The HNCIP included a test of ability to do housework as well as paid work – the implication being that if a married woman could earn her keep from her husband by doing housework, she should be his responsibility for maintenance, not the State's. The ICA debarred married women from entitlement on the grounds that 'they would be at home anyway' (i.e. married women needed no compensation for earnings forgone as a result of providing high levels of assistance to a disabled person) (McLaughlin, 1991). Under the impact of the 1979 Equal Treatment Directive both the HNCIP and the ICA have been reformed – the HNCIP and NCIP were replaced in 1983 by a single Severe Disablement Allowance, which made no distinction between claimants on the grounds of marital status; and the ICA was extended to married women in 1986 (consequent on the Drake case taken to the European Court).

However, despite the removal of overt discrimination, women remain discriminated against when they are carers or disabled because they are disproportionately likely only to be eligible for non-contributory benefits rather than contributory benefits and hence to receive lower incomes. Originally non-contributory benefits were set at 60 per cent of the level of contributory benefits 'in order to maintain a preference for contributors' (McLaughlin, 1991), and the gradual downgrading of contributory insurance benefits under Conservative policy has led to some levelling of non-contributory relative to contributory benefits. However as Table 8.2 shows, non-contributory benefits continue to occupy the lowest ranks of the social security system and fairly substantial differences in rates continue for example, compare the £36.60 ICA with the £48.25 unemployment benefit or the £61.15 retirement pension. It was precisely these kinds of comparisons which led the Social Security Advisory Committee to say of the 1986 Social Security Review:

> We do not think the present proposals have taken adequate account of women's non-financial contribution to the economy and we

Table 8.2   Men's and women's benefit levels, £ per week, 1996–97

	Per week	
	Claimant	Adult dependent
Men's benefits		
1. Industrial Injuries Benefits:		
Disablement benefit 100% assessment	99.00	
2. Retirement pension	61.15	36.60
3. Incapacity benefit		
lower rate under pension age	46.15	
higher rate under pension age	54.55	
long-term rate	61.15	36.60
4. Statutory sick pay	54.55	
5. Unemployment Benefit	48.25	29.75
Women's benefits		
6. Maternity allowance:		
lower rate	47.35	
higher rate	54.55	
7. Income support		
Single adult	47.90	
Adult couple	75.20	
8. Severe Disablement Allowance	36.95	21.95
Age-related additions		
high	12.90	
middle	8.10	
lower	4.05	
9. Invalid Care Allowance	36.60	21.90
10. Child Benefit	10.80 (1st child)	
	8.80 (2nd + child)	

believe a further review is required to ensure that the benefit system applies fairly both to men and to women.

No such further review took place and neither is one on the current political agenda.

The importance of the assumptions in the social security system that mothers, and by extension all adult women, are exclusively engaged, or ought to be so, in unpaid caring work in the home, that any paid work they do is peripheral 'pin money', and that married or cohabiting women can look to men for financial support, is greater than such material comparisons imply. As ideological constructs they have a cultural import, and are also part of more general policies and provisions (for instance, in the social care field, see Dalley, 1988) which may push women into, or keep women in, unwelcome family forms and unwelcome relationships, as well as being responsible for unpaid caring work ('informal care') into which they are drawn with varying degrees of reluctance or enthusiasm (Finch and Groves, 1983; Finch and Mason, 1993; Graham, 1983, 1993; Land and Rose, 1985; McLaughlin, 1991; McLaughlin and Glendinning, 1994; Ungerson, 1983, 1987). However, it has also been the social security system which has allowed many women to leave unwelcome family relationships – and it is to this that the next section turns.

Lone motherhood

Although Beveridge failed to obtain agreement for the introduction of insurance benefits for divorced and separated women, women, whether mothers or not, have been able to claim means-tested benefits in their own right if they establish an independent household, and as lone mothers to claim such benefits without being available for paid work until their youngest child is 16. During the 1960s, 1970s and 1980s, lone motherhood increased steadily. The number of divorces per 1,000 married people rose from 2.1 in 1961, to 6.0 in 1971, 11.9 in 1981 and 12.8 in 1988, while the number of births outside marriage as a percentage of total births rose from 8.4 in 1971 to 12.8 in 1981 to 25.6 in 1988 (Lewis, 1995, p. 39). While there is some evidence that the divorce rate may now be stabilising, and that divorces involving children may even be falling, the proportion of births taking place outside of marriage has continued to grow – to 27 per cent in 1989, to 31 per cent in 1992 (Land, 1994, p. 95). The easing of conditions for divorce in the 1960s, the introduction and improvement of domestic violence legislation in the 1970s and 1980s, the reduction of the stigma attached to 'illegitimacy' and less favour towards adoption, were all given practical meaning for women by the existence of means-tested benefit support. That is, what might otherwise have been the 'empty promise' of, say, domestic violence legislation, became the possibility of independent living through the use of benefits to support women's own decisions about with whom, and how, they wished to live. These wider developments coincided with an increased emphasis on the right of people in need to claim means-tested benefit when the National Assistance system was reformed in 1966 to become the Supplementary Benefit (later the Income Support) system. Although the main objective was to encourage retired pensioners with little besides their state insurance pension to claim, the attitudes of other groups of claimants were affected too (Land, 1994, p. 94; Lewis, 1995, p. 40). As Land puts it:

> Thus although not easy, living on means-tested benefits was not so much worse than struggling on a low wage in the absence of adequate child care or living with a husband who was unable or unwilling to provide adequate support.
>
> (1994, p. 94)

This is not to suggest that the availability of benefit support created a 'dependency culture' with hordes of mothers, with the co-operation of fathers, opting for hand-outs from the state rather than participation in the labour market, or that it made fathers 'unnecessary'. Studies of lone mothers have repeatedly shown that if as many lone mothers had been engaged in paid work as said they wished to be, the proportion in employment would be similar to two parent families (Lewis, 1995). And the absence of a father continues to mean substantial economic insecurity and poverty for mothers and children. As Falkingham and Hills (1995, p. 136) point out, those who are observed as poor in any one year may not be poor on a lifetime basis (for example, those in full-time education can be 'temporarily poor' but lifetime rich). However, their analyses show that lone parenthood is associated with both annual and lifetime poverty:

> Moving up through the lifetime income distribution: the proportion of women falls; age-at-death tends to rise … lone parenthood falls; the proportion experiencing divorces falls for women but rises for men …Women who experience five or more years as a lone parent have much lower incomes than those who marry but are

never divorced. By contrast men who divorce emerge as a well-off
group in late middle-age.

(Falkingham and Hills, 1995, pp. 136, 106–107)

Notwithstanding the financial penalties that accrue to women as a result
of lone motherhood, it is true that 'To a considerable extent assistance-
based benefits permitted a substantial transformation of the family.
Women with children and without men were able to live
autonomously, albeit not well' (Lewis, 1995, p. 45).

It was precisely this transformation – what Conservative politicians
thought of as the inadvertent nationalisation of fatherhood (Land,
1994), and what feminists would describe as a shift from private to
public forms of patriarchy – that the recent Child Support Act seeks to
redress: '[it seeks to] put this particular genie back in the bottle and
fundamentally to change the pattern of support of lone mother families
away from the state and towards men and lone mothers themselves'
(Lewis, 1995, p. 45).

The Child Support Act (1991)

As Millar (1994a) points out, three factors came together to make the
introduction of the new arrangements for the support of lone mothers
and children a priority for the Conservative government. First, a rising
public expenditure bill, for example, from £1.4 billion in 1981 to £3.2
billion in 1988–89 (Land, 1994, p. 92), much of which was attributed to
the decline in receipt of maintenance among lone parents. In 1979, half
of all lone parents receiving state benefits were also receiving maintenance but by 1989 this had fallen to 23 per cent. Despite the
government's assumption that this was due to an increasing unwilling-
ness among fathers to pay, both the National Audit Office and the
House of Commons Public Accounts Committee attributed the decline
in maintenance payments in part at least to the reduction in resources
the DSS was spending on recovering maintenance (through the 'liable
relative' officers whose job it was to track down absent fathers) during
the 1980s (ibid., p. 96). A further factor was the operation of the
Matrimonial and Family Proceedings Act 1984 which ended the life-
long obligation in common law for husbands to maintain their wives,
permitting husbands and wives the option of a one-off settlement
instead. Land (ibid.) reports that during the 1980s the courts did indeed
encourage once-and-for-all property settlements in which a husband
gave up claims on the matrimonial home in return for lower or no
maintenance to the ex-wife who was caring for their children.

There were two other more general impetuses, however: the ideology of the (patriarchal) family – that is, that absence of the father is 'bad for society', leading to crime, unemployment, and so forth; and the ideology of a welfare dependency culture – that is, that those on benefits (whether mothers, present or absent fathers, or others) were too ready to rely on welfare handouts rather than taking responsibility for themselves. On the one hand, this general anti-welfare thrust implied the enforcement of participation in the labour market, but to treat lone mothers as primarily market workers raised difficult issues for conservative values about gender roles and specifically motherhood. Treating lone mothers as workers first and mothers second might for instance have led other mothers to expect to be treated the same, leading to demands for public support for childcare and 'family-friendly' employment legislation (Millar, 1994a), and would thereby begin to undermine the idea(l) of the male family wage. On the other hand, there was no ambivalence about a father's role – that was to be a breadwinner. The specific provisions of the CSA thus ended up emphasising fathers paying instead of the state, with a little, but not too much, encouragement for lone mothers to take paid work in order to 'kill as many as three birds with one stone' (ibid.).

Given such ambivalence, it is not surprising that the CSA and associated changes in social security provision were confused about encouragement to lone mothers to take paid work. First, no attempt was made to counteract the discouragement (already strong, see previous section) for those with childcare costs to combining part-time employment with receipt of benefits following the Social Security Act 1986, when the (small) amount which could be earned without affecting the level of income support (which replaced supplementary benefit) was calculated on gross earnings instead of, as previously, net of travel and childcare expenses (Land, 1994, p. 95). Second, it was not seen as appropriate to provide publicly funded childcare and therefore a rather clumsy mechanism of disregarding some kinds of childcare costs for the purposes of the calculation of family credit was introduced. This required mothers to use childcare providers who could produce valid receipts (in other words, the more expensive forms of childcare) but the amount which could be disregarded was low in relation to the costs of substitute care for pre-school children in particular. Initially £40 a week could be disregarded, yielding a potential net gain of £28 (McLaughlin, 1994a). The inadequacy of this approach has led to the disregarded amount being increased to £60 a week from 1996–97. Third, the maintenance formula used by the CSA controversially included an amount for 'the parent as carer' (£44 a week at the time of introduction), in addition to the amounts for children, which could continue until the youngest child was 16 – an age well beyond that which prevents a mother from taking paid employment – leading to speculation (by absent fathers) that some 'vengeful' ex-wives would deliberately stay out of employment so as to force the absent father to pay as much as possible for as long as possible.

There was, however, no such ambivalence about enforcement of a duty on biological fathers to support their children (although as Eekelaar (1991) pointed out, the primary obligation seems to be in relation to the state rather than the child, since the amount payable in maintenance is a proportion of assessable income irrespective of the number of children). The Act also seems to introduce a new responsibility to maintain mothers. Absent fathers are not only obliged under the CSA to maintain their children – an obligation firmly rooted in centuries-old common law – but, as pointed out above, also the mothers, as carers of their children, irrespective of their marital status.

> The government denies that this represents a break with the past but the father of a child born outside marriage has not previously been under any duty to support the mother. Indeed in Victorian times it was thought to be very undesirable for a woman to have any claims on a man for maintenance, even for her children, unless she was married to him.
>
> (Land, 1994, p. 97)

This new responsibility, together with the fact that the costs of supporting stepchildren in second families is ignored in the maintenance formula, supports an interpretation of the Act as primarily targeted at persuading men to reduce the number of children they beget through serial relationships, whether marital or otherwise. Lewis, though emphasising only those children produced from serial marital relationships, makes the same point:

> The goal of the policy seems to be to persuade men to have only as many children as they can financially support. This is in line with the New Right's emphasis on personal responsibility ... If the Agency's powers are fully exercised, then men may not feel free both to remarry and have more children. Whereas the Finer Committee felt that the impossibility of mounting an attack on this behaviour in a free society meant that the state had to shoulder the major part of the burden of financial support, the current strategy does not accept this. It rejects rather than tries to reconcile the

historically accepted idea in public law that men support the families they live with, and in private law that they should pay something towards the families they have left; and it seeks instead to make them pay for both in so far as there are biological children present in both.

(Lewis, 1995, p. 43)

One of the chief problems with the Act is the degree of 'social engineering' it attempts. 'Natural' parental obligations are defined as absolutely unconditional when many people, men especially, do not regard their financial obligations (never mind care obligations) as unconditional (Burgoyne and Millar, 1994; Clarke *et al.*, 1993). Rather, these obligations tend to be seen as conditional on several factors: which partner was 'to blame' for the marital break-up; whether the absent father has the kind of access he wants to the children and often the ex-partner as well; and whether impregnation was accidental or intended. Thus the 1990 British Social Attitudes survey, for example, found that although 90 per cent of men and 95 per cent of women thought absent parents should pay maintenance, only 51 per cent thought this should continue if the caring parent remarried, while 13 per cent said it should stop and 33 per cent thought continued maintenance should be conditional on the new partner's income. Precisely because provision of maintenance is often thought of as conditional on access to the woman as well as the children by fathers, some 11,000 lone mothers have stopped claiming Income Support because, say campaigners, they want to avoid contact with violent fathers (Land, 1994) and as the CSA goes back through long-standing cases in which no maintenance is being paid, this group can be expected to grow.

Problems in the operation of the Child Support Agency, as well as disagreement with some of the principles embodied in the maintenance formula in the Act, have led to an active and vocal campaign against it (see Land, 1994 for further detail). Operational issues such as the high proportion (about half) of cases wrongly assessed; and the targeting of fathers with straightforward financial affairs first and/or those who were already paying some, but not enough, maintenance (rather than those paying none); together with some reports of absent fathers experiencing disincentives in relation to paid employment (Clarke *et al.*, 1993), were the primary factors behind the House of Commons Social Security Committee's (which examines the expenditure, administration and policy of the Department of Social Security and its associated public bodies) examination of the Agency's operations in 1993. Following its report in December 1993, some aspects of the formula were modified and a further review of the Agency's work was announced in April 1994. Despite considerable attention, reviews and reforms, however, a number of problems – tending to be those which affected, or might affect, mothers and children more than fathers – have had little airing.

To take children first, some children may see their fathers less often, or not at all, since expenses connected with visiting children, or having children visit, were ignored in the formula, which poses particular problems for those living a considerable distance away from their children, whose access costs can easily run into several hundreds of pounds per year, if not more. As a result some fathers after an assessment may decide that they can no longer afford to maintain contact with their children (Land, 1994, p. 98). Similar disregard to the needs of children is evident in two other aspects of the Act. First, whereas the Children Act (1989) puts the welfare of child(ren) paramount in any decisions concerning where and with whom they live and have contact in the event of a family breakdown, the Child Support Act only requires that their welfare be taken into consideration (ibid., pp. 92–93). Second, children in second families, whether stepchildren or biological children, will be at increased risk of poverty, since their needs are not taken into account by the formula.

As regards women, the fact that the Act ignored 'clean break settlements' (in which fathers gave up their share in the equity in the matrimonial home or borrowed money in order to secure a home for their former wife and children in return for reduced maintenance payments) and that this generated a lot of publicity, may make it more difficult to secure agreements that women and children can remain in the marital home following marital breakdown in future. The emphasis on biological fatherhood in the child support arrangements, already referred to above, involves a further 'sexualisation' of the administration of social security akin to that in relation to cohabitation discussed earlier. If an initial response by a man to a Child Support Agency enquiry results in him disputing parentage, the Agency returns to the lone mother with enquiries such as: when and where the relevant sex act took place; how often the woman had sex with the man in question; whether contraceptives were used; the date of the woman's last period before the contested impregnation; and whether the woman had sex with anyone other than the alleged father in the last three months before conception. Interestingly, none of these intrusive and intimate questions are actually of any use in determining parenthood. The Child Support Agency will almost certainly have to take men disputing fatherhood to court, and at that stage a DNA test will almost certainly be required. Land (1994) reports that about 1,000 women are now involved in difficult paternity suits, and suggests that this will rise in the future.

Finally, and most importantly for women, children and poverty, the Act has, and will, result in increased insecurity and risk of poverty. The Act's purpose is to have more of women and children's incomes derived from individual men rather than the state, but the state has only gone so far as to insist that a standardised maintenance amount is calculated. There are no guarantees for women and children that the maintenance calculated will actually be paid by absent fathers, and only very long-drawn-out mechanisms are available to women and children to enforce payment of maintenance. In contrast, the Finer Committee, and many other commentators since, have argued that the only method which would not increase the vulnerability of women and children is a Guaranteed Maintenance Scheme, in which the State pays the mainte-nance to the women and children and then recovers it from the absent father. The current UK approach – to leave it to the absent father to pay the maintenance direct to the woman and children – inevitably renders women and children more dependent on men (Millar, 1994a). It is clear that the ability and purpose of the social security system to address/redress primary poverty have been compromised by this latest attempt to use the social security system to promote and enforce partic-ular forms of familial relationships.

Social security reform and welfare regimes

The feminist approach to social security has involved documentation of the higher incidence of poverty amongst women (and children) than men, a redefinition of poverty, drawing out of the assumptions about gender roles that underpin provision, and analysis of the benefits of social security provision for women, however limited and incomplete. In recent years, feminists have also challenged mainstream ways of evalu-ating, comparing and theorising welfare regimes in different countries, particularly the use of the concept of de-commodification as a both a way of categorising and evaluating different welfare regimes. Coined by Esping-Andersen (1990), de-commodification refers to the extent to which welfare states weaken an individual's market dependence. However, in its original formulation, the concept did not acknowledge the very different ways men and women connect to the market (i.e. how, historically, men and women have been 'commodified' to different extents in the labour market), nor did the approach as a whole recognise the equally different ways men and women have been positioned in the family (McLaughlin and Glendinning, 1994). Thus, while 'dependence' on market work is assumed to be something men would be better off without, market work has empowered some women from excessive dependency in the family, including the ability 'to exercise a basic civil right to leave an oppressive relationship, literally to vote with their feet' (Hobson, 1994, p. 171). But it has not only been market work which has empowered women in this way – as this chapter has shown, under certain circumstances, social security provision may do likewise. As a result, a number of writers have proposed different ways of attempting to capture the positive and negative effects particular combinations of the 'market-and-family' in welfare regimes may have for women.

Lewis (1992) proposed a set of criteria for constructing social policy regimes based upon their degree of attachment to a male breadwinner/family wage ideology, since this is the most visible and coherent expression of specific market–family configurations across countries. In terms of assessing the value of different welfare regimes for women, O'Connor (1993) argued for supplementing de-commodification with a concept of non-dependency in personal life, insulation from personal and public dependence as well as from labour market pressures; while Orloff (1993) suggested the use of a generic concept of independence, assessing individuals' freedom from compulsion to enter potentially oppressive relationships in a number of spheres. Similarly, Lister (1994) and McLaughlin and Glendinning (1994) suggested the use of a concept of familism and its counterpart de-familialisation, to refer to the degree to which welfare regime 'packages' provide freedom from compulsion to enter or remain in oppressive family relationships, and/or their capacity to transform the power bases of familial relationships. As these new approaches to the assessment of welfare regimes develop and mature, they should begin to provide ways to judge the relative merits of proposals for reform of the current UK social security system. Already they serve to remind us that reforms to one part of a welfare regime alone (e.g. the social security system) may not have the extent or kind of impact desired by those proposing them. Further, they suggest that the 'benchmark' for reforms should be the extent to which they would enhance individuals' autonomy across the public and private divide.

In the UK, proposals to reform the social security system tend to fall into two main groups – those who argue for a change in the unit of entitlement for means-tested benefits from the couple/family to the individual and those who argue for substantial reform of the contribution and benefits sides of the National Insurance system, so as to include those undertaking part-time market work and those undertaking unpaid work. In addition some of those in both camps argue for the introduction of benefits for carers, such as a parental care allowance. Pushed to its limits the first approach encompasses those supporting the introduction of Basic Income (for example, Parker, 1993); while pushed to its limits, the second approach encompasses those supporting a Participation (or Citizens) Income (for example, the Commission on Social Justice, 1994). There is insufficient space here to discuss the details or relative merits of such proposals. All of them would be 'expensive' – one estimate of individualisation was that it would cost the equivalent of seven pence in the pound on income tax (Hills, 1993), while estimates of the taxation implications of fully fledged Basic Income rise to as much as double the current rate of income tax on additional income. Reform through extension of the insurance system would probably be somewhat less expensive and could be introduced more gradually. Whether such 'expense' is worth it, of course, depends on the value attached to the development of fiscal systems which redistribute income from men to women to a greater extent than the present one does, and/or which offer people freedom not only from material poverty but also enhanced autonomy and substantial change in the balance of power in familial as well as market relationships.

References

Alcock, P. (1993) *Understanding Poverty*, London: Macmillan.

Beveridge, W. (1942) *Social Insurance and Allied Services*, Cmnd 6404, London: HMSO.

Bradshaw, J. and Millar, J. (1991) *Lone Parent Families in the UK*, London: HMSO.

Burgoyne, C. and Millar, J. (1994) 'Child Support: the views of separated fathers', *Policy and Politics* 22(2): 95–104.

Callendar, C. (1995) 'Women and employment', in C. Hallett (ed.) *Women and Social Policy: An Introduction*, London: Prentice-Hall/Harvester Wheatsheaf.

Clarke, K., Craig, G. and Glendinning, C. (1993) *Children Come First? The Child Support Act and Lone Parent Families*, Manchester: Barnados, the Children's Society, NCH, NSPCC and SCF.

Commission on Social Justice (1994) *Social Justice: Strategies for National Renewal*, London: Vintage Press.

Dalley, G. (1988) *Ideologies of Caring: Rethinking Community and Collectivism*, London: Macmillan.

Davies, H. and Joshi, H. (1994) 'Sex, sharing and the distribution of income', *Journal of Social Policy* 23(3): 30–40.

Deacon, A. (1995) 'Spending more to achieve less? Social security since 1945', in D. Gladstone (ed.) *British Social Welfare: Past, Present and Future*, London: UCL Press.

Deacon, A. and Bradshaw, J. (1986) 'Social security', in P. Wilding (ed.) *In Defence of the Welfare State*, Manchester: Manchester University Press.

Eekelaar, J. (1991) *Regulating Divorce*, Oxford: Clarendon Press.

Esam, P. and Berthoud, R. (1991) *Independent Benefits for Men and Women*, London: Policy Studies Institute.

Esping-Anderson, G. (1990) *The Three Worlds of Welfare Capitalism*, Cambridge: Polity Press

Evandrou, M. and Falkingham, J. (1995) 'Gender, lone-parenthood and lifetime income', in J. Falkingham and J. Hills (eds) *The Dynamic of Welfare: The Welfare State and the Life Cycle*, Hemel Hempstead: Prentice-Hall.

Evason, E. (1991) 'Women and poverty', in C. Davies and E. McLaughlin (eds) *Women, Employment and Social Policy in Northern Ireland: A Problem Postponed?*, Belfast: Policy Research Institute.

Fairbairns, Z. (1985) 'The cohabitation rule – why it makes sense', in C. Ungerson (ed.) *Women and Social Policy: A Reader*, London: Macmillan.

Falkingham, J. and Hills, J. (eds) (1995) *The Dynamic of Welfare: The Welfare State and the Life Cycle*, Hemel Hempstead: Prentice-Hall.

Finch, J. and Groves, D. (eds) (1983) *A Labour of Love: Women, Work and Caring*, London: Routledge & Kegan Paul.

Finch, J. and Mason, J. (1993) *Negotiating Family Responsibilities*, London: Routledge.

Glendinning, C. and Millar, J. (eds) (1987) *Women and Poverty in Britain*, Hemel Hempstead: Harvester Wheatsheaf.

Glendinning, C. and Millar, J. (eds) (1992) *Women and Poverty in Britain: The 1990s*, Hemel Hempstead: Harvester Wheatsheaf

Graham, H. (1983) 'Caring: a labour of love', in J. Finch and D. Groves (eds) *A Labour of Love: Women, Work and Caring*, London: Routledge & Kegan Paul.

—— (1987) 'Being poor: perceptions and coping strategies of lone mothers', in J. Brannen and G. Wilson (eds) *Give and Take in Families*, London: Allen & Unwin.

—— (1993) 'Feminist perspectives on caring', in J. Bornat, C. Pereira, D. Pilgrim and F. Williams (eds) *Community Care: A Reader*, Basingstoke: Macmillan.

Hills, J. (1993) *The Future of Welfare: A Guide to the Debate*, York: Joseph Rowntree Foundation.

Hobson, B. (1994) 'Solo mothers, social policy regimes and the logics of gender' in D. Sainsbury (ed.) *Gendering Welfare States*, London: Sage.

Land, H. (1983) 'Poverty and gender: the distribution of resources within families', in M. Brown (ed.) *The Structure of Disadvantage*, London: Heinemann.

—— (1994) 'Reversing "inadvertent nationalisation of fatherhood": the British Child Support Act 1991 and its consequences for men, women and children', *International Social Security Review* 3–4/94: 91–100.

Land, H. and Rose, H. (1985) 'Compulsory altruism for some or an altruistic society for all?', in P. Bean, J. Ferris and D. Whynes (eds) *In Defence of Welfare*, London: Tavistock.

Lewis, J. (1995) *The Problem of Lone Mother Families in Twentieth Century Britain*, STICERD, Welfare State Programme Paper WSP/114, London: LSE.

—— (1992) 'Gender and the development of welfare state regimes', *Journal of European Social Policy* 2(3): 159–173.

Lister, R. (1992) *Women's Economic Dependency and Social Security*, Manchester: Equal Opportunities Commission.

—— (1994) ' "She has other duties": women, citizenship and social security', in S. Baldwin and J. Falkingham (eds) *Social Security and Social Change: New Challenges to the Beveridge Model*, Hemel Hempstead: Harvester Wheatsheaf.

McCay, N., Trewsdale, J. and McLaughlin, E. (1999) *Women's Incomes and the Social Security System*, Belfast: Equal Opportunities Commission.

McKay, S. and Marsh, A. (1994) *Lone Parents and Work*, London: HMSO.

McLaughlin, E. (1991) *Social Security and Community Care: The Case of the Invalid Care Allowance*, London: HMSO.

—— (1992) 'Introduction: towards active labour market policies', in E. McLaughlin (ed.) *Understanding Unemployment*, London: Routledge.

—— (1994a) *Flexibility in Work and Benefits*, London: IPPR/CSJ Issues Paper No. 11.

—— (1994b) 'The demise of the institution of the job', *The Political Quarterly* 65(2): 179–190.

McLaughlin, E. and Glendinning, C. (1994) 'Paying for care in Europe: is there a feminist approach?', in L. Hantrais and S. Mangen (eds) *Concepts and Contexts in International Comparisons: Family Policy and the Welfare of Women*, Cross-national Research Papers, Series 3, No. 3, Loughborough: Centre for European Studies, University of Loughborough.

McLaughlin, E., Millar, J. and Cooke, K. (1989) *Work and Welfare Benefits*, Aldershot: Avebury.

McLaughlin, E., Trewsdale, J. and McCay, N. (1999) *Women Excluded from National Insurance*, Belfast: Equal Opportunities Commission.

Marsh, A. and McKay, S. (1993) *Families, Work and Benefits*, London: Policy Studies Institute.

Metcalf, H. (1992) 'Hidden unemployment and the labour market', in E. McLaughlin (ed.) *Understanding Unemployment*, London: Routledge.

Millar, J. (1993) 'The continuing trend in rising poverty', in A. Sinfield (ed.) *Poverty, Inequality and Justice*, Edinburgh: New Waverley Papers, University of Edinburgh.

—— (1994a) 'State, family and personal responsibility: the changing balance for lone mothers in the UK', *Feminist Review* 48, Autumn, 24–39.

—— (1994b) 'Lone parents and social security policy in the UK', in S. Baldwin and J. Falkingham (eds) *Social Security and Social Change: New Challenges to the Beveridge Model*, Hemel Hempstead: Harvester Wheatsheaf.

—— (1995) 'Women, poverty and social security', in C. Hallett (ed.) *Women and Social Policy: An Introduction*, London: Prentice-Hall/Harvester Wheatsheaf.

Novak, T. (1988) *Poverty and the State*, Milton Keynes: Open University Press.

O'Connor, J. (1993) 'Labour market participation in liberal welfare state regimes – issues of quantity and quality', paper presented at the International Sociological Association RC 19 Conference on Comparative Research on Welfare States in Transition, September 1993, University of Oxford, Oxford.

Orloff, A. (1993) 'Gender and the social rights of citizenship: the comparative analysis of gender relations and welfare states', *American Sociological Review* 58(3): 303–328.

Pahl, J. (1980) 'Patterns of money management within marriage', *Journal of Social Policy* 9(3): 313–335.

—— (1989) *Money and Marriage*, London: Macmillan.

Parker, H. (1993) *Citizen's Income and Women*, BIRG Discussion Paper No. 2, London: Citizens' Income.

Pascall, G. (1986) *Social Policy: A Feminist Analysis*, London: Tavistock.

Squires, P. (1990) *Anti-Social Policy*, Brighton: Harvester Wheatsheaf.

Ungerson, C. (1983) 'Women and caring: skills, tasks and taboos', in D. Gamarnikov, D. Morgan, J. Purvis and D. Taylorson (eds) *The Public and the Private*, London: Heinemann.

—— (1987) *Policy is Personal: Sex, Gender and Informal Care*, London: Tavistock.

Vogler, C. and Pahl, J. (1993) 'Social and economic change and the organisation of money within marriage', *Work Employment and Society* 7(1): 71–95.

Williams, F. (1989) *Social Policy: A Critical Introduction*, Cambridge: Polity Press.

9 'Race', social security and poverty

Gary Craig

Introduction

This chapter examines the contribution of social security benefits to alleviating poverty amongst Black and ethnic minority communities (henceforward 'Black communities'). The first section briefly reviews evidence of the growth of poverty amongst Black communities. Next the (limited) evidence about Black communities' experience of the social security system is examined, including use of 'cash-for-care' benefits. The evidence indicates that we know very little, relative to our knowledge of the experience of white claimants, about the experience of Black claimants. The final sections suggest why this may be so, concluding that institutional and individual racism has very significant effects on the ways in which cash benefits are structured and delivered and that the effects of these processes are compounded by the dimension of 'race' being missing from much research and policy discussion. Parts of this chapter draw on a longer argument published elsewhere (Craig and Rai, 1996).

That an adequate picture is lacking of the needs and experiences of Black communities in what is often described as a multi-racial society, can be illustrated by the following examples: first, a relatively recent UK text covering 'inequalities, opportunities and policies' from a 'race' perspective contains only one reference to social security benefits and that to an article then six years old (Braham *et al.*,1992). Second, an authoritative account of models of benefit take-up, while reviewing issues such as stigma in considerable detail, has virtually nothing to say on the subject of 'race', either in relation to past or future research (Craig, P., 1991). And, third, a 'comprehensive' study of *Britain's Black Population*, subtitled *Social Change, Public Policy and Agenda* (Luthra, 1997) has no reference to social security at all.

Poverty and Black communities[1]

Between 1977 and 1991, the number of people living in poverty, defined as less than half average income, rose from three million to 11 million (DSS, 1993a) with the poorest tenth of the population no better off than in 1967, while the richest 5 per cent had increases of almost 60 per cent since 1979 alone (Jenkins, 1994). At the same time, new policy measures, including those introduced by the New Labour government, have increasingly restricted eligibility for many benefits. The 'restructuring' of benefit provision (usually resulting in the replacement of certain benefits by others of more limited scope and generosity) has further emphasised the role of means-tested and discretionary benefits within the state sector and private income-replacement provision outside it, and led to a reduction in the real value of certain key benefits. These measures have been accompanied by highly publicised, ideological allegations of widespread fraud and inappropriate claiming. Taken together these factors are moving the social security system towards being a 'last-resort safety net' through which increasing numbers of claimants are wholly or partially slipping. Within this dismal context, the ability of the social security system to maintain Black households at reasonable income levels must seriously be questioned, particularly given the widespread and long-standing accusations against the system of at best, indifference to the needs of Black communities and, at worst, institutional racism.

Remarkably, neither the DSS nor the Agencies created under the Next Steps 'revolution' (Ditch, 1993), have in place a credible ethnic monitoring system. The Agencies operate, as the DSS did before them, a system of benefits delivery incorporating no coherent strategy of racial equality, whose 'colour-blindness' is mitigated only by certain provisions at the margins. As a result, targeted and large-scale research aimed at exploring the specific experience of Black communities is virtually impossible to execute. It is still not unusual for relatively experienced research teams to go into the field, not knowing the ethnic origin of respondents, not being able to draw a sample based on ethnic origin, and having little idea as to whether translation or interpretation facilities are necessary or whether the design of research instruments incorporates an appropriate understanding of the cultural and social contexts of respondents. Similarly, the official DSS annual review of data (DSS, 1993b) provides no analysis based on ethnic origin. We may find within it a gender-based analysis of the length of spells on sickness benefit, for example, or the age distribution of households in receipt of community charge benefit, but not the ethnic origin of claimants or their household members in either case. The more recent Family Resources Survey

(DSS, 1995), of incomes of a 'representative sample of households in Great Britain', does include some information about benefit take-up by members of Black communities but, as the Survey report itself acknowledges for much of the relevant data, 'care should be taken in interpreting the figures because of the small sample sizes' (ibid., p. 6). The Rowntree *Inquiry into Income and Wealth* also noted that 'ethnic minority incomes tend to be lower than those of the rest of the population' (Barclay, 1995, p. 28) but again, because data are drawn from surveys which do not focus on ethnicity, detailed analysis on this basis is not possible. More recently, drawing on both the Family Resources Survey and the Fourth National Survey of Ethnic Minorities (Modood *et al.*, 1997), Berthoud (1998) has argued that Pakistanis and Bangladeshis are 'four times as likely to be poor as white people. This arises for four reasons in combination: high male unemployment, low female economic activity, low pay, large families'.

The continuing opposition of successive Secretaries of State to ethnic monitoring (in a tacit alliance with social security trade unions) effectively precludes much useful 'race'-related social security research from being undertaken. Opposition amongst the unions is understandable given the fears existing since the mid-1980s (Gordon and Newnham, 1985), now shared amongst, *inter alia*, solicitors and fire(wo)men, that ethnic monitoring might be used to support an oppressive immigration regime. Nevertheless, it is difficult to see how, without ethnic monitoring carried out under suitable operational arrangements (for example, within the context of an independent statistical service) adequate, reliable information about the circumstances of Black communities can be assembled. Particularly given the continuing difficulties in introducing even a single, widely accepted 'ethnic' Census question, the prognosis is not encouraging for those exploring policy issues to do with the impact of 'race' on the delivery and receipt of social security benefits.

This is alarming because, as Amin and Oppenheim's review (1992) of Black communities' experience of poverty demonstrates, there are key structural factors increasing the likelihood of Black communities experiencing poverty, compared with the population as a whole. These include higher than average and relatively increasing unemployment levels, resultant both on Black communities' concentration in inner city areas where older industrial sectors have borne the brunt of recession and the international restructuring of capital, and the racist way in which people are selected for jobs or made redundant (TUC, 1994, 1995); their greater likelihood of working in low-paid jobs, a result also of more wide-ranging racial discrimination; more limited access to adequate and appropriate health (Nazroo, 1997) and housing provision (e.g. 53 per cent of registered homeless in London are Black); and the increasing restrictions on the ability of refugees and asylum seekers to access help from the social security system.

Given this greater risk of poverty, it should fall to the social security system to provide both a more general compensatory mechanism for maintaining adequate income levels, and also a means to identify Black communities at greatest risk. However, Amin and Oppenheim identify further factors which, far from allowing the social security system to achieve these functions, effectively undermine its ability so to do. The most significant of these, compounded by a lack of adequate data, are:

- the emphasis within remaining contributory schemes on non-interruptions of contributions, which militates against the position of those who cannot maintain steady contributions because of irregular earnings, short working lives in the UK, and absences abroad (Patel, 1990);
- the consequent over-reliance of such groups on means-tested benefits, notorious for low take-up levels as a result of a range of factors including ignorance, poor information and individual or structural racism (e.g. for Family Credit recipients, take-up of free dental care for ethnic minority claimants was recently estimated at 44 per cent: for white claimants it was [still the very low] 62 per cent);
- direct and indirect discrimination through conditions placed on 'people from abroad', such as sponsorship, residence and 'public funds' tests (for example, eligibility for Severe Disablement Allowance requires residence in the UK for 10 of the 20 years prior to a claim); and
- direct and indirect discrimination and racism in the administration and delivery of social security benefits, including the failure to provide adequate translation and interpretation services. In Youth Training Schemes, for example, membership of which was a condition for receipt of Income Support (IS) between the ages of 16 and 18, adequate provision was not made for the cultural and religious needs of some young Asian women (Craig, G., 1991; Maclagan, 1992).

Social security cash benefits are also of increasing importance in relation to debates about the financing of community care.[2] These debates have focused largely on questions of overall resources and only more recently on the issue of 'who pays?', that is, on the extent to which carers and users of care services could contribute to the costs of care, to the exclusion of discussion of the role of social security in meeting individual care needs. Constraints on overall resources, combined with the maintenance of traditional 'top-down' modes of service delivery, continue to exclude all but the most determined user groups from participation in the planning and delivery of care services (Craig, 1993). These constraints create even greater barriers to Black communities, barriers which may be exacerbated by the development of private care markets. These are unlikely to meet the needs of small, unpopular or poor groups of service users, or of those whose needs may be more difficult to identify. The needs of poor Black care users are thus likely to be marginal to most provision (Craig, 1992a, 1993): those attempting to make use of care-related benefits may be doubly disadvantaged.

More likely to be poor?

Five and a half per cent of the UK population (roughly three million people) are members of Black communities, including 1.6 per cent black (including black-Caribbean, black African and black 'other'), 2.7 per cent South Asian (mainly Indian, Bangladeshi and Pakistani) and 1.2 per cent Chinese and 'others'. This Black population lives mainly in or near large English cities such as Birmingham, London, Bradford, Leicester and Manchester (Owen, 1992). Almost two-thirds of all Black communities live in areas characterised by traditional manufacturing industry and in parts of central and inner London (ibid.), areas where, as noted earlier, there has been significant restructuring of local employment opportunities leading to unemployment, under-employment or low-waged employment amongst Black communities. Labour Force Survey data show that compared with a 'white' unemployment rate of 7 per cent in 1989–90, the corresponding rate for black-Caribbeans was 14 per cent, for Pakistanis 22 per cent and for Bangladeshis 25 per cent. By 1993, the position had deteriorated: compared with an unemployment rate of 5 per cent amongst the white population, the rates were 25 per cent for black populations and 30 per cent for Pakistanis and Bangladeshis (Sly, 1994).

There are also significant variations by age and gender: for example, the peak unemployment rate for Pakistanis is in the age range 16–24, whereas for Bangladeshis it is in the 45–64 range (Jones, 1993). An analysis of ethnicity and gender in the West Midlands Labour Force (Andersen, 1993), based on the 1991 census, suggests that the unemployment rate for economically active Pakistani females in the West Midlands was 42.5 per cent compared with 7.5 per cent for white females. Seventy per cent of 16–24-year-old Blacks in London are unemployed.

The household and age structure of different Black groups are diverse and this also has implications for the structure and use of different social security benefits. Thus, for example, about 60 per cent of South Asian families comprised couples with children, twice the rate for white and black families (Owen, 1994). On the other hand, proportionately about four times as many Black families comprise lone parent families as for white or South Asian families. This has implications for the ethno-centric assumptions underpinning the Child Support Act about family structure and parental responsibilities which have yet to be addressed.

At the other end of the age spectrum, although one-sixth of the white UK population was aged 65 and over in 1988, the Black communities with the highest proportion of 65+ members were the Indian and black-Caribbean groups at only 3 per cent (FPSC, 1991). While there is some evidence that access to informal carers is markedly greater amongst some Black groups than in the UK population as a whole (Wilmott, 1986), there are grounds for concern regarding Black elders' access to income. Given the lower level of educational qualifications achieved by members of Black communities while in the labour market, their shorter employment careers while in the UK, and greater likelihood of unemployment and low pay, Black pensioners are more likely to have both reduced access to occupational pensions, and reduced state pensions and other contributory benefit provision. Their income is thus likely to be lower than that of their white counterparts (Jolley, 1988).

Although the inter-relationship of gender and race has yet to be explored in any detail, we know that the position of women from Black communities is particularly precarious in relation to eligibility and access to social security benefits (Cook and Watt, 1992). Female economic activity rates are higher for black-Caribbean women than for women in general and almost four times as high as for South Asian women. However, black-Caribbean economically active women are only slightly more likely to work full-time than women of South Asian origin, and both groups are far more likely to work full-time than white women. Black-Caribbean households are far more likely to be dependent on just a woman's wage than white households, but because of what Lister (1992) describes as the 'gender-blind' nature of poverty statistics, it is not easy to map the extent to which the social security system responds adequately to the differing economic and social situations of Black families. Lister's review indicates that Black women are over-represented amongst the low paid and the unemployed, and, as is now well known, that women in general are more vulnerable to poverty than men. Although social security statistics do not provide consistent analyses on the basis of gender, it is also clear that women's access to contributory benefits is much lower than men's. Yet again, however, although take-up of some pre-pension age benefits (particularly, for example, Family Credit, Severe Disablement Allowance and Invalid Care Allowance) is dominated by women, we know virtually nothing about the extent to which the dimension of race affects the take-up patterns of such benefits.

For those Black groups whose overall demographic profile is 'younger' than that of the UK population as a whole, dependence on income-replacement (especially means-tested) social security benefits will be higher than that of the general population. For 'older' Black groups, especially Bangladeshis and Pakistanis, benefit issues, as we have seen, are coming to be concerned with retirement and other pensions, and non-retirement but 'post-employment' benefits, including the range of care-related benefits referred to again below. Access to, knowledge and delivery of benefits are therefore correspondingly more significant issues for Black claimants. What, then, do we know about Black communities' experience of the social security system?

'Race' and social security provision: recent research findings

Remarkably, prior to a relatively recent small-scale research project (Bloch, 1993), there is little evidence that the Department of Social Security regarded the issue of Black access to social security as a serious focus for research at all. Indeed, the then DHSS, in one early evaluation of social security administration and delivery, attempted to suppress the publication of findings which revealed a significant level of overt and indirect racism amongst DHSS officials (Cooper, 1984). This disregard for the 'race' dimension began to be corrected even outside the DHSS only from the mid-1980s.

For example, the Third Policy Studies Institute Survey (a large-scale quantitative study) into 'the circumstances of the British black population' (Brown, 1985), covering the question of household income within a brief section on 'support and care', noted the relatively very small proportion of pensioner-only households amongst Black households and the varying – but generally higher – levels of dependence on key social security benefits (especially unemployment benefit, Child Benefit and supplementary benefit) amongst Black groups, compared with the white population. The study revealed that Black respondents felt they were treated worse than white respondents by the social security system. The low level of policy and research interest in and knowledge of 'race' issues in relation to social security was also reflected in a Bibliography published at the time (Gordon and Klug, 1983). Compared with 66 entries under 'Citizenship and Nationality' (itself part of a very extensive section on immigration and nationality), there were only 14 entries under 'welfare rights' and no separate 'social security' section at all (although there were 47 entries under 'social services').

Although the DSS appears more open now to discussion about the needs of Black communities, the level of official disinterest, apparently based on this 'colour-blind approach', during the 1980s and early 1990s, is in marked contrast to the attention paid to the needs of Black communities in some other areas of social policy, for example, the developing debates about ethnicity and health (Bhopal, 1997), or what Harrison (1993, p.2) refers to as the 'startling development towards ethnic pluralism ... in the social housing field'. Prior to Bloch's study, it has been left almost entirely to individual academics and to the voluntary sector to raise even limited questions about the ability of Black communities to access social security or the appropriateness of DSS responses to their needs.

From the mid-1980s, research into the experience of black claimants falls into four broad categories in terms of the auspices of the study. First, small-scale, sometimes anecdotal, research based on the work of local community organisations (e.g. Mahtani, 1992; Tarpey, 1984). Second, reports synthesising wider-ranging sources of information on specific race-related issues to do with social security benefits, delivery and administration (e.g. Amin and Oppenheim, 1992; Gordon and Newnham, 1985; NACAB, 1991). Third, more general research accounts (based either on small-scale qualitative or large-scale survey research) of social security issues which incorporate a specific focus on Black communities' experiences (Becker and Silburn, 1990; Cohen *et al.*, 1992; Craig, 1989; Finch, 1990; Huby and Dix, 1992; Marsh and McKay, 1993; Petch, 1994; Ritchie and England, 1985). This focus ranges from the incidental to the more central, but the studies characteristically, in the words of one researcher, make 'an effort to include people from different ethnic minorities'. Fourth, studies which have been targeted specifically on the experience of Black communities (Bloch, 1993; Law *et al.*, 1993; Sadiq-Sangster, 1991). Few of these reports were specifically commissioned or funded by the Department of Social Security. Key findings from these studies are reviewed below.

Gordon and Newnham (1985) synthesised evidence, largely in the form of case studies drawn from advice centres, relating to racism in the social security system. Their report observed 'little has been done to highlight the plight of one particular group of welfare claimants – black people – who ... are second-class claimants', commenting that the absence of research was 'surprising'. Where the position of Black people as claimants was examined, the 'problem' was defined as 'one of language and culture – for example, the absence of information translated into minority languages' (ibid., p. 2). This was, the authors concluded, certainly one problem but only a part of the 'racism which permeates the whole social security system' (ibid.).

Much of this report focuses on the connections between social security benefit entitlement, and issues of nationality and the control of immigration which as Walker and Ahmad (1994) observe, led to Black people ' being fearful of making claims to which they are fully entitled' (see also Skellington and Morris, 1992). It also reviewed the extent of institutional and individual racism within the social security system. By the time of its publication, the DHSS was in the process of translating key leaflets into major Asian languages although it had been less than assiduous in ensuring their effective distribution. The DHSS had also, at that time, only two offices where interpreters were officially employed 'in cases of special difficulty', relying instead in the remainder of its 400+ offices on claimants' 'younger family members and friends' to undertake interpretation.

One impetus for examining the 'Black' experience of social security came from the 1986 Social Security Act with its increased emphasis on discretionary and means-tested benefits (notably the social fund) (BRC, 1985). One early, largely descriptive commentary on the social fund in practice (Craig, 1989) reflected the concern that discretion based on notions of deserts would lead to discrimination against Black claimants. Independent evidence available at the time was anecdotal and ambiguous on this question (Becker and Silburn, 1990).

Discretion has historically had an important place within the social security system. Although its scope may give the appearance of generosity, the local practice of discretion may deny this (Adler and Asquith, 1981). Discretion allows for political adjustments in the face of uncertain situations and thus provides a mechanism both for the rationing of benefits and for the classification of claimants in a way which is obscure but which works to the disadvantage of those groups regarded by the state as the 'undeserving' poor (Craig, 1992b). Given the often-contested status as citizens and nationals of members of Black groups, in the context of increasing controls on immigration (such as have been developing for some time), it has not been difficult for politicians concerned with limiting public expenditure, tacitly to characterise black claimants as 'undeserving' and 'scroungers' (Golding and Middleton, 1982; Gordon and Newnham, 1985). The impact of general ideological attacks on so-called 'undeserving' claimants are particularly significant for members of Black communities given their physical visibility because of skin colour.

However, despite widespread concern about the impact of increased reliance on discretion, researchers conducting the DSS-funded official evaluation of the social fund, based on a mix of qualitative and quantitative methodologies, were not required to focus particularly on the needs of Black claimants nor consequently were able to provide any separate 'race'-based assessment of the fund's impact (Huby and Dix, 1992). The only indication of a 'race' dimension in the study is a Technical Note stating that nine potential respondents out of 3,553 sample addresses were discarded because of 'language problems'. Cohen *et al.* (1992) evaluated the more general impact of the 1986 Act, including within the two qualitative studies brought together in their report, a significant sub-sample of Pakistani (largely Mirpuri Muslim) claimants, interviewed in their language of choice by Pakistani interviewers. Both studies reported institutional racism, for example as a result of inappropriate assumptions about family and community life which were reflected in the day-to-day operation of the social fund, as well as incidences of individual racism within local DSS offices.

Additionally, the study carried out in Bradford (where restructuring of the textile industry had led to a rapid increase in unemployment amongst local Bangladeshi and Pakistani communities), suggested that the DSS had made little progress even in the provision of translation and interpretation facilities. The one interpreter in the office serving the large Pakistani community (one of the offices referred to in Gordon and Newnham [1985]) 'only wrote in English and translation into other written languages had to be carried out at another office' (Cohen *et al.*, 1992, p. 52). In 1989, the Secretary of State had previously noted, in response to a written question on 'measures undertaken by the DSS to assist ethnic minorities in claiming benefits', that there were only five (limited) measures then in place:

i   publication in seven languages other than English of the key leaflet *Which Benefit?*;
ii a free Urdu and Punjabi telephone helpline;
iii training courses for local office staff servicing multi-racial communities;
iv the interpreter and liaison service in Bradford; and
v   signs and posters in local offices and public areas.

(*Hansard*, 21 February 1989, col. 593)

This DSS response, however, was not only limited in terms of the remit of the Department itself, it also failed to address the impact of wider structural processes of discrimination.

Mahtani's (1992) Sheffield study is typical of a number of small-scale (and, in some cases, unpublished) investigations into wider policy issues facing Black communities. This examined problems of credit and debt (for both employed and unemployed people) within a local Pakistani community, again through semi-structured interviews conducted by locally recruited Pakistani interviewers. The study revealed a familiar contradiction: that respondents were in greater poverty and greater need, facing increased levels of debt compared with the population at large, yet made relatively low use of debt advice services: 'reasons advanced for not using advice services (including the DSS) included the difficulty of language, a lack of awareness of where to seek advice, and the feeling that an adviser from a different background would not understand the Pakistani culture nor the implications of their advice' (ibid., p. 37). The study recommended specialist debt advice workers for the Pakistani community, better translation and publicity provision and better training and information for all parties involved in local debt and credit work.

The report provoking the most significant response from the DSS to date was *Barriers to Benefit* (NACAB, 1991). The Citizens' Advice Bureau (CAB) service had increasingly dealt with queries from Black users during the 1980s, recruiting black and Asian advisers in response to this trend, and social security was one of its two major ongoing areas of advice work (accounting for about 1.8 million queries or 24 per cent of all enquiries in 1992–93). NACAB had intermittently reported on issues related to the needs of Black communities (Cowell and Owen, 1985; GLCABs, 1986; NACAB, 1984) but this report represented their first major national public statement on the experiences of Black claimants. It was based, typically for national NACAB reports, on an analysis of a substantial number of cases focused on defined topics, culled from the information returns of almost 100 (self-selected) local bureaux.

The report's most substantial conclusions were that racism was common in the social security system and that 'black clients and clients who speak or write no or little English are not receiving full entitlement to benefit and their encounters with the social security system are often distressing and humiliating' (NACAB, 1991, p. 2). This arose, NACAB concluded, because the DSS 'refuses to accept responsibility for people who do not understand DSS communications in English' (ibid.). NACAB recommended that the DSS should give a clear commitment to racial equality, and to improving its performance in terms of different language forms, translation and interpretation facilities, the images used in publicity material, training and support for those working with Black claimants: a familiar checklist.

One significant outcome of the NACAB report was the agreement of the DSS to establish liaison arrangements with NACAB in order to monitor developments. In 1993, NACAB's informal soundings with local bureaux suggested that 'there had been good local initiatives in some areas but that overall there was still a long way to go'. By that time, however, the Benefits Agency had been established to administer benefit delivery and committed itself in writing to 'providing services fairly and impartially, never discriminating on any grounds including those of race, sex, religion or disability'. A further indirect outcome of the pressure generated by NACAB's work was that the DSS commissioned a small study on the information needs of Black communities.

This study (Bloch, 1993) mainly comprises 101 'semi-structured interviews with customers and potential customers from six linguistic groups' (ibid., p. 4), representative of different lengths of residence, religious affiliations and first languages. The (again familiar) recommendations arising from the study were that local offices of the Benefits Agency 'develop a deeper understanding of the communities they serve', consult with local community groups, hold benefits surgeries, improve translation and interpretation facilities and recruit more staff from Black communities. It was also recommended that further research be undertaken, particularly through a large-scale survey 'to obtain more detailed and statistically representative data' (ibid., p. xiii) about claiming patterns. The report does not suggest how an appropriate sampling frame could be constructed. Significantly, when asked what their most useful source of information had been about social security provision, respondents most often mentioned local advice workers, friends or relatives.

Two other studies, Law et al. (1993) and Sadiq-Sangster (1991), investigate attitudes to claiming social security benefits among Black communities. In the former, five different Black communities were selected to examine their attitudes to claiming. The findings identify key factors contributing to low benefits take-up: the administrative complexity of the benefit system; the inaccessibility of the Benefits Agency (e.g. perceived difficulties of communication with Benefits Agency staff); and religious and cultural factors such as a sense of stigma attached to claiming, based on a belief that those who claim would be looked down on in the community. The study demonstrated the simultaneous impact of these dimensions on benefit take-up. Among the Bangladeshi community, Law et al. found that the sense of stigma, particularly among young people, was based on reasons enshrined in the Islamic laws of self-sufficiency and autonomy achieved through work. Many younger Bangladeshi respondents only claimed benefit after exhausting all alternative avenues, in contrast with older people having a work history in this country. The latter reconciled claiming benefit, based on a contributory system, with the Islamic model of contributing to collective funds to help the poor and needy.

The late claiming factor was also noted by Sadiq-Sangster (1991), in a study of Pakistani Mirpuri families. She examined not only the impact of religious beliefs, but also the lack of adequate help in making claims, finding that some families had consequently accumulated serious debts. Her study showed that stereotyped assumptions about close Asian family support systems are often misconceptions. This kind of support was on occasions not available to some families, not necessarily because it was not wanted, but because either there was no extended family nearby or members of the extended family were in equally difficult situations. Sadiq-Sangster illustrates the family support and reliance system which is based on a complex system of tradition involving '*lena-dena*', or exchange of functions, providing direct material goods or indirect support incurring costs (e.g. visiting and caring for sick relatives, attendance at sibling weddings). Inability to fulfil these functions can seriously affect family relationships and the perceived and expected dependency on family support. These expenditure patterns, reflecting essential elements within the lifestyles of community members, are not acknowledged within the social security system. Sadiq-Sangster's study also illustrates how the experiences of individual Black claimants at Benefits Agency offices affect their take-up of benefits.

The most recent report on difficulties experienced by Asian claimants (CRE, 1995) also pointed to the impact of racism. Claims made by Asian people took longer to process than other claims; supporting evidence was required more often for Asian claims (even though non-Asian claimants more often provided inadequate information); and Fraud Officers were more often drawn in, usually inappropriately, to examine Asian claims for benefit, than for other claimants.

As noted above, the issue of cash benefits for community care purposes is becoming an important area of debate and we conclude this part of the discussion by briefly considering aspects of this issue. The major social security benefits relevant to this discussion are Income Support and the relevant premiums, together with the social fund; non-means-tested/extra costs benefits such as Attendance Allowance (AA), Disability Living Allowance (DLA), Invalid Care Allowance (ICA),

Invalidity Benefit (recently replaced by the more restricted Incapacity Benefit) and Severe Disablement Allowance; and contributory benefits such as retirement pensions and sickness and unemployment benefits.

The literature on the 'race' dimension of 'cash-for-care' issues is also sparse. A comprehensive literature review of 'community care in a multi-racial Britain' (Atkin and Rollings, 1993) contains only one reference to social security benefits within its index. A short section on the financial burdens of care, which notes that 'black people ... are further disadvantaged because their incomes are likely to be lower than those of white people' (ibid., p. 17) refers only to six published sources. One database does exist as a result of the large-scale surveys of disablement by the OPCS, commissioned by the DHSS to inform its review of disability benefits. These surveys (e.g. OPCS, 1988) found that the rates of disability for 'Asians' and 'West Indians' (OPCS classifications) were 12.6 per cent and 15.1 per cent, respectively, compared with 13.7 per cent for 'whites'. This database does not, however, appear to have been further utilised to explore benefit issues for Black communities nor have the DSS' more well-funded explorations of 'cash-for-care' issues (e.g. McLaughlin, 1991) had an explicit 'race' dimension.

One small-scale survey (McFarland et al., 1989), indicates how even issues of access to care benefits become 'overlooked' within Black communities. None of the 60 respondents identified welfare rights as a problem area: only 28 per cent of the sample mentioned the DHSS as a useful source of help and considerably fewer knew of other potential places to seek advice (such as the local Social Work Department and even the Community Relations Council). The need for a 'major welfare rights ... campaign, utilising material in the main community languages, thus emerged very strongly' (ibid., p. 411). The issue, the researchers felt, was not limited needs but 'barriers of awareness and communication'.

Figgess et al. (1993) highlighted some of the barriers to be surmounted by Black communities in their analysis of the development of effective local services for people with disabilities. The postal survey, sent to a sample of those in receipt of selected disability benefits, achieved a good overall response rate but a very low representation (4 per cent of all respondents, less than half their local representation as a whole) from Black communities. The survey, which reviewed the take-up of benefits, reported, echoing the findings of earlier studies (e.g. Barker, 1984; CIO, 1988; ADAPT, 1993), the need for leaflets in languages other than English.

The promotion of benefits take-up is a major issue to be faced by local authorities which are now being drawn, frequently reluctantly, into the development of community care charging regimes as a result of constraints on community care funding from central government. Indiscriminate charging arrangements are open to the accusations that they particularly penalise poorer clients/care-users or, where they attempt to 'claw back' disability benefits such as AA or DLA, that they effectively make disabled care users pay twice for services, both through council tax and a charge. Many local authorities are developing charging policies at the same time as attempting to construct strategic responses to the growth of poverty in their areas (Alcock *et al.*, 1995). The Association of Metropolitan Authorities has attempted to develop a coherent charging policy for local authorities which tries to square the circle between the principle that 'user pays' is fairer than spreading the cost of services across all local authority residents, and the recognition that most social services provision is used predominantly by those in receipt of social security benefits.

Here again, members of Black groups may be most vulnerable since the adoption of means-tested charging schemes, favoured by many local authorities, is likely to impact negatively on users' attitudes to services. The AMA acknowledge (AMA/LGIU, 1992) that Black claimants, because of under-claiming, may not be entitled to concessionary 'passporting' schemes for free service use but, to date, suggests only that effective benefit checking systems should be put in place as part of care assessment processes. Clearly, if local authorities had adequate ethnic minority records – which most don't (NISW, 1991) – they could at least plan focused take-up campaigns for specific benefits. Small-scale studies (Jadeja and Singh, 1993) also reflect on both the impoverishment of Black Elders and ways in which charging policies which take no account of 'race', will disproportionately affect them.

'Race': the marginal dimension in research

However, the detailed findings of the recent study by Rai (1995) demonstrate how racism percolates quite specifically into the research process itself. This study aimed, *inter alia*, to identify the range of research practices for conducting qualitative social research among Asian communities. One of its central findings was that where a research organisation has no specialist role in addressing the 'race' dimension in research, it is dependent on the interest of individual researchers to include 'race' issues in research. On rare occasions, the funders or commissioners of research may specify consideration of 'race'-related issues in research studies. However, Rai found, in a culture where research agendas are set by funding bodies in consultation with the research community, 'race' overall tends to be invisible. An absence of organisational policy, strategy or practice ethos to address the 'race' dimension thus inevitably results in *ad hoc* and inconsistent practice patterns.

Rai also notes that the low proportional representation of Black communities in the population as a whole is often used to justify their exclusion from general research designed to have wider applicability. It is believed that research that addresses Black communities incurs high costs and requires complex research designs. The supposed high costs tend to be associated with the collection of data in relevant community languages. Methodologically, in quantitative research, it is argued that the low numbers of potential respondents from Black communities lead to statistically insignificant results. The use of booster samples is often viewed as an unsatisfactory solution, mainly on the grounds that these require complex research designs with the need to carry out complicated and costly analysis. Also there are reservations about using current sampling techniques for Black communities. Researchers argue that samples drawn only from densely populated 'Black' areas are not representative and biased against members of these communities who live elsewhere. In qualitative research, it is believed that low numbers of members from Black communities in small sample sizes lead to meaningless data and results. Researchers interviewed by Rai also reported a lack of knowledge on how to address 'race' in research, citing uncertainty about which Black communities to include in particular studies, and a lack of awareness of their specific cultural norms and social circumstances. A 'play safe' option is adopted, resulting in ignoring Black communities in research.

Against these arguments, which reflect the dominant practice, Rai found that the few specialist organisations and interested individual researchers engaged in 'race'-related research, observe the position of UK Black communities from a perspective based on their real circumstances and experiences. These researchers recognise that Black communities often face the severest social problems, for example higher levels of unemployment and a higher level of dependency on state benefits, as demonstrated earlier. They also note the methodological limitations, for example of the sampling techniques available for Black communities as discussed above.

However, instead of these limitations resulting in a dismissive response on 'pure' statistical grounds, Rai argues that the social context of Black communities living in concentrated urban areas gives rise to specific problems – such as high unemployment, poverty, lack of adequate housing – which need to be addressed accordingly. Some official databases indeed calculate the density of ethnic minority populations as indicators in the assessment of levels of deprivation (DH, 1992). Those problems of a methodological nature that are cited as reasons for not addressing Black communities in research, thus have in these cases to be handled as complexities that have to be addressed with an acceptance that high costs may be incurred.

Rai concluded that the resulting emphasis on cultural and linguistic issues, which characterises much social research touching on the experience of Black communities, continues to perpetuate their problematisation and marginalisation. Problems experienced by Black communities remain 'invisible', except in rare instances, for example, those studies which draw attention to structural discrimination in the social security system, and the discriminatory treatment of Black communities by some social security staff, providing some explanations for the low benefit take-up among these communities. The findings of studies such as those by Law *et al.* (1993), Sadiq-Sangster (1991) and, to a lesser extent, Cohen *et al.* (1992) are important as they highlight specific problem areas which are generally overshadowed in other research studies focusing on linguistic and cultural differences, and which sometimes inadvertently contribute to common perceptions of 'ignorant' Black communities. In fact, it is the limitations of the latter studies themselves which provide us with an incomplete picture. The emphasis within them remains on looking for the source of problems among Black communities: other crucial structural findings largely remain hidden.

Conclusion

Clearly, any identifiable information needs of Black communities revealed by more limited research should not be disregarded. However, the focus on these kinds of issues alone, prevalent in what continues to be a limited range of 'race'-related social security research studies, is problematic. Without a critical approach to addressing the 'race' dimension in social policy research along the lines outlined above, most studies will continue at least partially to obscure some of the real causes of social problems amongst Black communities, and problematise the members of those communities themselves. Additionally, without an adequate national system of ethnic monitoring of social security customers, independent of political interference, we cannot effectively examine the extent, nature and consequences of the low benefit take-up amongst Black communities. All the evidence from small-scale studies, as we have shown, points to the very great scope of this problem on a national scale. The causes and incidences of institutional and individual racism within the social security system remain largely to be addressed, although the action needed has to be situated in a wider programme of social, political and economic action.

So-called 'multicultural' social security policy is at present seriously flawed, the costs in terms of financial and social citizenship being borne most of all by those least responsible for those flaws. The evidence summarised here suggests both that members of Black communities are not receiving income to which they are entitled and that they are structurally disadvantaged in their treatment by the social security system. This impacts on other important areas of citizenship, such as their prospects for receiving and purchasing effective and appropriate social and health care. The greatest challenge for the social policy community is that much current research fails to demonstrate the structural reasons for this state of affairs.

Notes

1 Sections 2 and 5 draw in parts on the work of Amin and Oppenheim (1992), and Rai (1995), to each of whom the author is considerably indebted.
2 A fuller discussion of this issue can be found in Craig (1992a) and Glendinning and Craig (1993).
3 The findings of the Fourth National Survey of Ethnic Minorities (Modood *et al.*, 1997) appeared too late to be incorporated adequately into this analysis.

References

ADAPT (1993) *Asian and Disabled*, Bradford: Spastics Society/Barnados.

Adler, M. and Asquith, S. (1981) *The Politics of Discretion*, London: Heinemann.

Alcock, P., Craig, G., Dalgleish, K. and Pearson, S. (1995) *Combating Local Poverty*, Luton: Local Government Management Board.

AMA/LGIU (1992) *A Review of Issues Relating to Charging for Community Care Services*, London: Association of Metropolitan Authorities/Local Government Information Unit, mimeo.

Amin, K. and Oppenheim, C. (1992) *Poverty in Black and White*, London: Child Poverty Action Group/Runnymede Trust.

Andersen, H. (1993) *Ethnicity and Gender in the West Midlands Labour Force*, Birmingham: West Midlands Low Pay Unit.

Atkin, K. and Rollings, J. (1993) *Community Care in a Multi-racial Britain*, London: HMSO.

Barclay, P. (1995) *Income and Wealth*, vol. 1, York: Joseph Rowntree Foundation.

Barker, J. (1984) *Black and Asian Old People in Britain*, London: Age Concern UK.

Becker, S. and Silburn, R. (1990) *The New Poor Clients*, Nottingham: Nottingham University Benefits Research Unit/Community Care.

Benefits Editorial (1994) 'Race, racism and social security', *Benefits*, Issue 9. Nottingham: January, p. 1.

Berthoud, R. (1998) 'The incomes of ethnic minorities', paper to Seebohm Rowntree Centenary Conference, University of York, March.

Bhopal, R. (1997) 'Is research into ethnicity and health racist, unsound or important science?', *British Medical Journal* 314, 14 June, 1751–1756.

Bloch, A. (1993) *Access to Benefits*, London: Policy Studies Institute.

Braham, P., Rattansi, A. and Skellington, R. (eds) (1992) *Racism and Anti-Racism*, London: Sage/Open University.

BRC (1985) *The Social Security Reforms*, London: British Refugee Council.

Brown, C. (1985) *Black and White Britain*, London: Policy Studies Institute.

CIO (1988) *Double Bind*, London: Confederation of Indian Organisations.

Cohen, R., Coxall, J., Craig, G. and Sadiq-Sangster, A. (1992) *Hardship Britain*, London: CPAG.

Cook, J. and Watt, S. (1992) 'Racism, women and poverty', in C. Glendinning and J. Millar (eds) *Women and Poverty in Britain: The 1990s*, Brighton: Harvester Press, pp. 11–23.

Cooper, S. (1984), *Observations in Supplementary Benefit Offices*, London: Policy Studies Institute.

Cowell, R. and Owen, S. (1985) *Ethnic Minorities and the CAB Service*, London: National Association of Citizens' Advice Bureaux.

Craig, G. (1989) *Your Flexible Friend?*, London: Social Security Consortium/Association of Metropolitan Authorities.

—— (1991) *Fit for Nothing?*, London: COYPSS/Children's Society.

—— (1992a) *Cash or Care: A Question of Choice?*, York: Joseph Rowntree Foundation.

—— (1992b) 'Managing the poorest', in T. Jeffs *et al.* (eds) *Changing Social Work and Welfare*, Buckingham: Open University Press.

—— (1993) *The Community Care Reforms and Local Government Change*, Hull: University of Humberside Social Research Papers No.1.

Craig, G. and Rai, D.K. (1996) 'Social security, community care – and "race": the marginal dimension', in W. Ahmad and K. Atkin (eds) *'Race' and Community Care*, Buckingham: Open University Press.

Craig, P. (1991) 'Costs and benefits', *Journal of Social Policy*, 20(4): 537–566.

CRE (1995) *The Provision of Income Support to Asian and Non-Asian Claimants*, Manchester: Manchester Commission for Racial Equality

DH (1992) *Key Indicators of Local Authority Social Services*, London: Department of Health/HMSO.

Ditch, J. (1993) 'Next Steps: restructuring the Department of Social Security', in R. Page and N. Deakin (eds) *The Costs of Welfare*, Aldershot: Avebury, pp.64–86.

DSS (1993a) *Households Below Average Income*, London: Department of Social Security, HMSO.

—— (1993b) *Social Security Statistics 1993*, London: Department of Social Security, HMSO.

—— (1995) *Family Resources Survey Great Britain 1993/4*, London: Department of Social Security.

Dutt, R. and Ahmad, A. (1990) 'Griffiths and the Black perspective', *Social Work and Social Sciences Review* 2(1): 37–44.

Figgess, S. *et al.* (1993) *Information Survey Report*, Oldham: Oldham Disability Alliance/University of Oxford, mimeo.

Finch, H. (1990) *Perspectives on Financial Support for the Elderly*, London: SCPR.

FPSC (1991) *An Ageing Population*, London: Family Policy Studies Centre.

GLCABS (1986) *Out of Service*, London: Greater London Citizens' Advice Bureaux.

Glendinning, C. and Craig, G. (1993) 'Rationing versus choice', in R. Page and N. Deakin (eds) *The Costs of Welfare*, Aldershot: Avebury, pp. 165–182.

Golding, P. and Middleton, S. (1982) *Images of Welfare*, Oxford: Martin Robertson.

Gordon, P. and Klug, A. (1984) *Racism and Discrimination in Britain*, London: Runnymede Trust.

Gordon, P. and Newnham, A. (1985) *Passport to Benefits*, London: Child Poverty Action Group.

Harrison, M. (1993) 'The Black voluntary housing movement', *Critical Social Policy* 39: 21–35.

Huby, M. and Dix, G. (1992) *Evaluating the Social Fund*, Department of Social Security Research Report No. 9, London: HMSO.

Jadeja, S. and Singh, J. (1993) 'Life in a cold climate', *Community Care* 22 April, pp. 12–13.

Jenkins, S. (1994) *Winners and Losers*, York: University of Swansea/Joseph Rowntree Foundation.

Jolley, M. (1988) 'Ethnic minority elders want more sensitive services', *Social Work Today* 14 January, p. 8.

Jones, T. (1993) *Britain's Ethnic Minorities*, London: Policy Studies Institute.

JRF (1995) *Inquiry into Income and Wealth*, York: Joseph Rowntree Foundation.

LASA (1985) 'Black claimants target for cuts', *Review* August, London: London Advice Services Alliance.

Law, I. *et al.* (1993) *Racial Equality and Social Security Service Delivery*, Leeds: School of Sociology and Social Policy, Research Working Paper No. 10, University of Leeds.

Lister, R. (1992) *Women's Economic Dependency and Social Security*, Manchester: Equal Opportunities Commission.

Luthra, M. (1997) *Britain's Black Population*, Aldershot: Arena.

Macfarland, E., Dalton, M. and Walsh, D. (1989) 'Ethnic minority needs and service delivery', *New Community* 15(3), April, pp. 405–415.

Maclagan, I. (1992) *A Broken Promise*, London: COYPSS/Youthaid/Children's Society.

McLaughlin, E. (1991) *Social Security and Community Care*, DSS Research Report No. 4, London: HMSO.

Mahtani, A. (1992) *Poverty, Debt and Indifference*, Sheffield: Sheffield City Polytechnic.

Marsh, A. and McKay, S. (1993) *Families, Work and Benefits*, London: Policy Studies Institute.

Modood, T., Berthoud, R., Lakey, J., Nazroo, J., Smith, P., Virdee, S. and Beishon, S, (1997)*Ethnic Minorities in Britain*, London: Policy Studies Institute.

NACAB (1984) *The Kirklees Ethnic Minorities Advice Project*, London: National Association of Citizens' Advice Bureaux.

—— (1991) *Barriers to Benefit*, London: National Association of Citizens' Advice Bureaux.

Nazroo, J.Y. (1997) *The Health of Ethnic Minorities*, London: Policy Studies Institute.

NISW (1991) *Ethnic Monitoring in Social Services Departments*, London: Race Equality Unit, National Institute for Social Work.

OPCS (1988) Report 1, *The Prevalence of Disability Amongst Adults*, London: HMSO.

Owen, D. (1992) *Ethnic Minorities in Great Britain*, Coventry: Centre for Race and Ethnic Relations, University of Warwick.

—— (1994) *National Ethnic Minority Data Archives 1991, Census Statistical Papers*, Coventry: Centre for Research in Ethnic Relations, University of Warwick.

Patel, N. (1990) *A 'Race' Against Time*, London: Runnymede Trust.

Petch, H. (1994) *The Bare Necessities*, London: CHAR/London Homelessness Forum.

Rai, Dhanwant K. (1995) *In the Margins: Social Research Amongst Asian Communities*, Social Research Papers No. 2, Hull: University of Humberside

Ritchie, J. and England, J. (1985) *The Hackney Benefit Study*, London: SCPR.

Sadiq-Sangster, A. (1991) *Living on Income Support: An Asian Experience*, London: Family Service Units.

Saggar, S. (1993) 'The Politics of "Race" Policy in Britain', *Critical Social Policy* 37: 32–51.

Skellington, R. and Morris, P. (1992) *'Race' in Britain Today*, London: Sage.

Sly, F. (1994) 'Ethnic groups and the labour market', *Employment Gazette* May.

Stubbs, P. (1993) '"Ethnically sensitive" or "Anti-racist"', in W. Ahmad, pp. 34–50.

Tarpey, M. (1984) *English Speakers Only*, London: Islington People's Rights.

TUC (1994) *Black Workers in the Labour Market*, London: Trades Union Congress.

—— (1995) *Black and Betrayed*, London: Trades Union Congress.

Walker, R. and Ahmad, W. (1994) 'Windows of opportunity in rotting frames?', *Critical Social Policy* 40: 46–69.

Wilmott, P. (1986) *Social Networks, Informal Care and Public Policy*, London: Policy Studies Institute.

10 Poverty and social security in the European Union

John Ditch

Introduction

There is a clear and ever more transparent European context to debates on poverty and social security in the United Kingdom. In part, this has emerged because of the United Kingdom's membership of the European Union but it is also due to a growing interest in comparative social policy as a basis for more imaginative policy-making. This chapter will address three questions: first, how does the UK's social security system compare with those of other countries in the EU? Second, what contribution has the EU made to reporting and reducing poverty levels? Third, what trends and challenges will shape the future of social security at a European level?

Historically, policy-makers in the United Kingdom have been slow to recognise the international context to questions about poverty, income distribution and social security. A rather complacent and, at times, smug belief that the United Kingdom was a world leader in providing high quality social security tended to reinforce an insular and detached approach to policy-making. The United Kingdom eschewed continental European models and examples, arguing that its historic and cultural ties were predominantly with the old Commonwealth of Australia, New Zealand and Canada. Even within this framework the tradition was, or so it was believed, that the UK represented the template to be followed across the world. Such a conception was as misconceived as it was arrogant. Not only had countries like New Zealand distinguished, deeply rooted and indigenous social security systems of their own but in many ways the old ties and trading relationships began to matter less as Britain slowly, and not without misgivings, re-oriented its economic and political gaze to Europe. In so doing, it became more apparent that the UK model, encoded by Beveridge and given lip-service by successive governments of both political persuasions, was not the only basis for income maintenance. Continental European countries had developed a contrasting model of social security, intimately linked to the principles and practice of Bismarckian social insurance, with implications for governance structures and the ranking of preferred social outcomes. An examination of the European context to social security must begin with a review of contrasting assumptions and vocabulary.

The most basic distinction between the UK and continental traditions of social security revolves around the social construction of cost and benefit. Whereas in the United Kingdom social security is generally regarded as a form of public support for the vulnerable and poor, on the continent of Europe there is a greater emphasis on transfer, reciprocity and solidarity. In the UK the emphasis is upon the strengths and weaknesses of allocative systems as they relate to individuals and families; in continental Europe the concern is with the societal context, the role of social security in the maintenance of stable, coherent, solidaristic communities. It is ironic, therefore, that continental systems are more based on an individual's relationship to the labour market in contrast to the UK system which has traditionally placed greater emphasis on citizenship status. In the former there has been more emphasis on social insurance compared with social assistance in the latter.

However, these historic differences (see Hills *et al.*, 1994) have, for the past two decades, begun to dissolve. This has been in part a process of spontaneous convergence and partly the planned outcome of policy initiative. The European Commission has argued (Quintin and Chassard, 1992) that, when compared to either American or Japanese alternatives, there is a coherent 'European model' which includes and conflates both Beveridgean and Bismarckian traditions: a gradual extension of minimum income provisions, on the one hand, and earnings-related income protection, on the other, with both approaches extended by a common and more vigorous commitment to so-called integration strategies. These come in two forms, positive and negative. The positive variant (diffusing from East to West) seeks to facilitate social (re)integration through programmes of training, life-long learning and sponsored employment; the negative variant (diffusing from West to East), seeks to establish activity within the labour market on the basis of tougher eligibility and conditionality rules for benefit entitlement. Demographic trends, labour market re-structuring and expenditure constraint are posing common challenges to all national social security schemes: the responses remain, however, remarkably diverse.

Just as continental European policy-makers and analysts tend to talk of social protection rather than social security, so there is a related, and distinctive, vocabulary which is slowly defusing into the English language. As will be elaborated in more detail below, the concept of poverty has given way to the wider construct of social exclusion and solidarity, cohesion and inclusion express some of the values which underpin conceptions of societal obligation and rights; *précarité* (precariousness) and exclusion describe the conditions which demand support and intervention.

These words are much more than devices for the representation of complex social processes, they become symbols which convey an orientation to social protection which is collective, corporatist and communitarian; the harsher and more restricted language code of Anglo-Saxon conceptions of social security place emphasis on individuals, dependency, incentives and behaviour. It is a complex and sometimes uncomprehending dialogue between continental and English-speaking traditions, made more difficult as a result of inconsistencies in translation, which mediates much of the growing struggle to reconcile contrasting approaches to remarkably similar challenges; the costs and consequences of unemployment, the costs and implications of ageing, the balance between competitiveness and social adequacy.

In contrast to countries in other parts of the world, continental European systems of social protection, like that of the UK, are broadly based and universal in character. All countries attempt, with varying degrees of coverage and success, to provide universal support to individuals and their dependants when in need. There has been a growing commitment to the extension of minimum income schemes across the whole of the EU (most recently in Portugal) consistent with the provisions of the 1992 Recommendations on minimum levels of income and social assistance (CEC, 1992b). Only Greece presently lacks any form of generalised social assistance scheme, though several others are rudimentary (Eardley *et al.*, 1996). Moreover, there is considerable variation not only in the generosity of assistance payments, the rules or conditions of eligibility, but also in the level of government responsible for their payments. Some schemes, of which the UK's Income Support is an exemplar, operate with (mostly) national rules and levels of benefits; others (as in Germany and France) operate via sub-national authorities, seeking to adapt social assistance to local circumstances and needs (Ditch *et al.*, 1997).

EU social security: an overview

Taking the mix of public and private, insurance and assistance-based schemes together, it is possible to group member states of the European

Union into four broad categories. The United Kingdom and Republic of Ireland share, in large part, a common language and to an extent which is sometimes overlooked, a common historical experience with respect to poor law and social insurance arrangements. The dominant pattern of health care is provided free at the point of consumption (though charges are remitted through a 'Voluntary Health Insurance' scheme in Ireland for those above a specified income level). Traditionally, and in both countries, insurance-based benefits have been flat rate and there has always been heavy reliance on the use of means-testing to select and support recipients.

The Scandinavian countries, Denmark, Sweden and Finland, share a distinctive and collective culture with an emphasis on high levels of social protection as a right of all citizens. There is, however, a history of firm emphasis being placed on re-integration and labour market programmes: generosity is tinged with firm expectations of job search or behaviour modification.

The continental European countries of Germany, France, Austria and Benelux, all have traditional Bismarckian systems. The key to social protection is provided by labour market status, and benefits are mostly earnings-related, with high replacement rates. There is a history of complex and rather distinct occupationally based systems which have been more recently supplemented by statutorily provided social assistance schemes.

The final group consists of the Mediterranean rim: Italy, Spain, Portugal and Greece. Social assistance schemes are very rudimentary and there is significant reliance on family and charities for support. There are sector and occupationally based insurance schemes and some can be generous. However, the totality of provision is inconsistent and highly fragmented.

European Union countries are, on average, among the world's high spenders on social protection. In 1995 expenditure (on social security and health care) averaged 28.5 per cent of EU GDP: over 4,800 ECU per person. The highest levels of expenditure are found in the Scandinavian countries and in The Netherlands (over 30 per cent of GDP), with the UK at 27 per cent, Portugal spending 20.7 per cent and Greece a little above 16 per cent. In per capita terms Luxembourg spends four times as much as Greece.

One of the big debates in the European Union over the past decade has concerned the impact of social protection on industrial competitiveness: long a concern of successive British governments, the position on the continent is made potentially more acute because revenue tends to come disproportionately from social insurance contributions, with employers being responsible for up to 60 per cent of these. The scale of 'non-wage labour costs' varies from country to country (but are especially high in France, Italy and Spain) but generally there has been pressure to shift the balance of contributions away from employers in favour of employees and the general tax-payer.

All social security systems cover the range of standard contingencies: old-age, employment, disability and sickness, maternity and family benefits. Financial support for older people takes the largest share of social protection in all countries (with the exception, just, of Ireland which has the youngest demographic profile in the Union) at around 45 per cent. Comparing the value of pensions is notoriously difficult: even allowing for the effects of differential purchasing power equivalents of national currencies, there are significant technical difficulties resulting from the multiple receipt of pensions and variation in retirement ages. For example, Italy commits a high proportion of GDP to pensions but the modest value of an individual pension reflects the low age of retirement which brings more claimants into the scope of eligibility. Research by Whiteford and Kennedy (1994) has underlined the importance of seeing pensions against the background of total transfer of resources to older people: cash benefits are but a part of the total package of resources which determine the relative standard of living of group in the population. Whereas the cash value of UK may be comparatively low, when health care, the value of housing and other 'freely' provided goods and services are taken into account, the resulting living standards of older people in the UK are relatively high.

The rise in the levels of unemployment has resulted in increased levels of expenditure through both insurance compensation and social assistance. In Belgium, Denmark, Italy and Luxembourg unemployment benefits are closely related to former income in work and are largely unrelated to either assets or savings. In contrast, in both the United Kingdom and Ireland over 60 per cent of unemployment compensation is means tested. A common theme is the extension of conditionality rules underpinning the move from so-called passive to active measures; however, despite emphasis on training and job-search measures, it is unclear whether these measures make a dent in the aggregate number of unemployed rather than act to 'churn' the balance between employed and unemployed (Eardley *et al.*, 1996).

Health care and sickness benefits, taken together, committed approximately 25 per cent of social protection expenditure in 1993. There has been an increase in the level of expenditure, partly a function of demographic ageing, the costs of advances in medical technology and partly due to the displacement effects of unemployment.

There has been a more varied pattern in respect of spending on invalidity, disability and industrial injuries benefits. Stable levels of expenditure in Belgium, Germany, France and Luxembourg have been matched by increased expenditure in The Netherlands and the United Kingdom. All across the European Union there has been downwards pressure on family and children's benefits for over a decade: expressed as a proportion of GDP, levels of expenditure have declined in most countries since 1989. The structure and value of support for families of different size, composition and income level varies greatly (for further details see Bradshaw *et al.*, 1993 and Ditch *et al.*, 1996).

Development of EU social security policy

The European Union, going back to its origins as a Common Market in the late 1950s, has a long-standing interest in social protection. During the negotiations leading to the Treaty of Rome (1957) the French government was keen to see measures included which promoted what was then called 'social harmonisation'. However, opposing arguments were vigorously advanced by the German government who were not persuaded that intervention in the field of social security was necessary to promote economic growth. As a result, there are some rather general statements contained in the Treaty about the need to address social security issues if by so doing the proper functioning of the market could be achieved. In particular Article 117 committed the signatories to the promotion of improved living and working conditions. Article 118 provided for closer collaboration in the social policy arena (including social security), but only at the instigation of member state governments.

In the late 1960s and early 1970s attention was paid to the need to regulate access and entitlement to social security benefits for migrant workers and their families. Building upon the provisions of Article 51 of the Treaty of Rome (which declared that workers should not be disadvantaged or penalised as a result of exercising their right to move freely within the European Economic Community), a new framework of European law has developed. Specifically, regulations No. 1408/71 and 574/72 require that there should be no difference in the treatment of nationals and non-nationals with respect to social security entitlements. The focus was, as it remains, very much upon the circumstances and rights of migrant workers and their dependants (Bolderson and Gains, 1993).

In 1986 the European Community, consistent with a broader awakening of concern about the 'social dimension', published a

Communication to the Council called *Problems of Social Security: Areas of Common Interest*. This document drew attention to a number of common trends of concern to all twelve member states of the Community. These concerns were grouped into three categories: first, financing problems resulting from the growing levels of reported disability and, second, 'demographic imbalance' which, it was argued, would result in unacceptable burdens on the European economy; third, there were problems associated with 'the new poor' – the young, lone parents and long-term unemployed, many of whom were inadequately supported under provisions of existing (and traditional) systems of social protection.

As will be seen below, there was growing evidence about the extent of poverty in the European Community and a (continental) commitment that the pursuit of a Single Market should not be achieved without regard to the circumstances of the most vulnerable and disadvantaged. Moreover, there was, in theoretical terms if not otherwise, a widespread belief that a Single Market should operate without facilitating or tolerating unfair competition; the prospects of 'social dumping' had been theorised and needed to be discounted in practice.

The Community Charter of Basic Social Rights for Workers adopted in 1989 by all member states (except the United Kingdom) led to the adoption of a Community Recommendation on the convergence of social protection objectives and policies in 1992 and to a Recommendation on common criteria concerning sufficient resources and social assistance in social protection systems (CEC, 1992a and 1992b). The United Kingdom argued that the interpretation of these Recommendations should take into account prevailing national social and economic circumstances. In the event, the UK government has had no difficulty meeting the conditions and expectations of the recommendations.

The European Community's quest for a human face, being a response to the costs of economic growth and linked to the accession of the United Kingdom, Denmark and Ireland had already resulted in the adoption of a Social Action Programme in 1974 which included provision for an anti-poverty initiative. The first European Community Programme to Combat Poverty covered the period 1975–80 but was extended to 1984: it had a very small budget of 20 million ECU and was mostly concerned with action-research projects (see Dennett *et al.*, 1982) aimed at identifying the dynamics of poverty at local level and the evaluation of pilot project to tackle its consequences. No less than nine national reports on poverty and anti-poverty programmes in the European Community were produced.

In 1983, as unemployment and the effects of the recession became more evident, a second 'Poverty 2' programme was approved by the Council of Ministers, covering the years 1986–89. This programme aimed 'to combat poverty more effectively and carry out positive measures to help the underprivileged and identify the best means of attacking the causes of poverty and alleviating its effects in the EC'. However, the budget was little improved: 20 million ECU was committed and the focus was once again upon small-scale action research demonstrations projects rather than large-scale intervention. In total, and across the EC, no less than ninety-one action-research projects were chosen by national governments and the European Commission for sponsorship.

A third ECPCP 'Poverty 3' (1990–94) was introduced following the reform of the Structural Funds in the late 1980s. The budget had been increased to ECU 55 million. On this occasion Eurostat was provided with funds to develop poverty indicators for cross-national comparisons, including the establishment of a household panel survey. In addition, an Observatory on Social Exclusion was established to monitor trends and policy initiatives (Room, 1995; Robbins *et al.*, 1994).

Against this background, the European Community has sponsored several enquiries and action programmes into poverty and its alleviation. In the mid-1980s it adopted a relative definition of poverty to determine the number living in poverty in Europe. Their definition was that: 'The poor shall be taken to mean persons, families and groups of persons whose resources (material, cultural and social) are so limited as to exclude them from the minimum acceptable way of life in the member state in which they live.' In empirical terms the EC poverty line was defined as 50 per cent of the mean disposable income in each country, adjusted for household size by means of the OECD equivalence scale. According to this definition some 30.5 million people were in poverty in 1980, compared to 38.6 million in 1975 and 43.9 million in 1985 (Jenkins and O'Higgins, 1989). In 1985, 14 million were unemployed, of whom one half had been out of work more than a year and a third for over two years. Thirty-five per cent of the jobless had never worked; no less than 3 million people were homeless.

Based on secondary analysis of family Budget Surveys Bardone and Degrys (1995) found (using the OECD equivalence scale and a poverty threshold of 50 per cent) that in 1988 some 14 per cent of households (approximately 17 million), equal to 16 per cent (approximately 52 million) people were poor in the EU. The implication is that larger families were more likely to experience poverty than smaller households. Adjusting the poverty threshold can make a significant difference to the reported levels of poverty. For example, reducing the threshold from 50 per cent to 40 per cent reduces the poverty rate from 14.6 per cent to 58 per cent of households in the United Kingdom. This would suggest that the 'poverty gap' (depth of poverty) in the United Kingdom is relatively weak (see Table 10.1).

Attempts to adopt a Poverty 4 programme have failed at the Council of Ministers because a number of member states (Germany and the UK in particular) have objected. One of the key changes to have occurred over the past decade has been the gradual movement away from a concern with 'poverty' to a concern with 'social exclusion'. Some member states have been reluctant to accept that poverty existed at all in

Table 10.1   Poverty rates by country according to the different poverty thresholds and equivalence scales at the end of the 1980s

In terms of:	OECD scale			Modified OECD scale			Subjective scale		
	40%	50%	60%	40%	50%	60%	40%	50%	60%
Household									
Belgium	1.9	6.1	13.7	1.7	6.6	14.1	3.6	8.3	17.5
Denmark	1.3	3.6	10.1	1.4	4.2	13.3	1.5	5.5	15.4
France	6.5	14.0	23.1	7.5	14.9	24.5	10.1	17.8	27.0
Germany	4.7	10.8	19.7	5.3	12.0	21.2	8.6	17.3	26.0
Greece	13.0	20.6	29.7	13.0	20.8	29.8	13.6	21.6	30.7
Ireland	8.4	16.9	27.0	7.9	16.4	26.9	11.8	20.0	28.6
Italy	11.2	20.6	30.4	12.5	22.0	32.2	14.8	24.8	34.3
Luxembourg	3.5	8.8	17.2	3.7	9.2	17.2	4.5	11.2	20.2
Netherlands	1.1	4.3	12.1	1.9	6.2	13.9	6.5	12.7	20.8
Portugal	15.7	25.2	34.4	17.3	26.5	35.2	20.2	29.2	38.0
Spain	8.6	16.7	26.2	9.3	17.5	27.1	12.9	21.2	30.6
United Kingdom	5.8	14.6	25.2	7.4	17.0	28.0	14.1	23.3	32.4
Person									
Belgium	3.0	8.6	17.7	2.2	7.4	15.5	2.0	5.6	13.2
Denmark	1.5	4.3	12.0	1.1	3.9	11.5	1.1	4.0	12.2
France	7.7	16.5	26.7	6.9	14.7	25.0	6.3	12.4	20.7
Germany	5.0	11.9	21.3	4.5	10.9	19.9	5.2	11.8	19.1
Greece	12.8	20.5	30.1	11.4	18.7	27.6	9.9	16.8	25.3
Ireland	10.1	19.4	30.3	7.5	15.7	26.3	6.5	13.0	20.7
Italy	12.0	22.0	32.3	11.6	21.1	31.4	11.0	19.9	29.2
Luxembourg	5.4	11.5	21.1	4.8	11.1	20.0	2.9	8.0	16.3
Netherlands	1.3	4.8	13.8	1.5	4.8	11.4	3.1	6.6	11.9
Portugal	15.5	25.1	34.6	15.5	24.5	33.3	14.2	22.3	30.5
Spain	9.2	17.7	27.7	8.7	16.9	20.0	8.6	15.7	24.4
United Kingdom	6.7	15.3	26.7	6.4	14.8	25.3	7.9	14.9	23.0

their countries, believing that it had been effectively eradicated by the functioning of social protection schemes. The concept of social exclusion is broader than income poverty but relates to participation and identity. However, the principle of subsidiarity, which accords precedence and policy-making responsibility to member states, means that the European Union does not have lead responsibility for eradicating social exclusion. That said, the Union's Structural Funds (Social Fund to help with labour market activities, Development and Cohesion Funds to support physical infrastructure in depressed regions, and the Common Agricultural Policy) all make a contribution to combating social exclusion but as a by-product of their primary objectives.

The phenomenon of social exclusion has increased significantly over the past decade or so. Homelessness has become more obvious, particularly in the large cities as have incidents of urban violence, ethnic tension and unemployment. There are indications that although fewer people experience long-term poverty, many more experience temporary bouts of poverty: what the French call *précarité*. This is linked to growth in numbers of lone parents.

Bardone and Degryse (1995) found evidence of a correspondence between high levels of social protection expenditure and low rates of poverty. There are two clusters of countries: on the one hand, are the Mediterranean countries, the UK and Ireland which have relatively low levels of social security spend and relatively high levels of poverty. On the other hand, France, Germany, Luxembourg, Belgium, Denmark and The Netherlands, by way of contrast, have higher spend and lower poverty. The correlation between spend and poverty is not so clear, however, within each group. For example, although The Netherlands has the highest spend, it is Denmark which has the lowest poverty level.

Bardone and Degryse conclude that 'social protection systems can, to varying degrees, help to reduce or prevent poverty, though this is not always the reason for which they were originally conceived'. Over the past decade, however, we have observed a shift away from the universal and insurance-based benefits in favour of means-tested, social assistance type, support. There has been greater emphasis upon specific populations groups (the unemployed, disabled or lone parents) or the development of a guaranteed minimum income available following a test of means. Guaranteed minimum income schemes were introduced in Luxembourg in 1986, in France (the RMI) in 1988 and in Portugal in 1996. Just as there are debates in the United Kingdom about the structure, funding and future of social security so there are at the European level. A recent Communication from the Commission (CEC, 1997) encapsulates the dimensions of debate.

A number of trends are placing new demands upon structures which, for the most part, were established over half a century ago. Changes in labour market structure, away from full-time, life-time employment in favour of flexibility pose a challenge to ensure that new forms of risk are covered by insurance and that longer-term entitlements can be built up. Linked to labour market change is the growth in female economic activity – both a product and a challenge for equal opportunities – which requires that social security systems allow for new forms of contribution and payment. Third, the continental European systems are much exercised by the implications of demographic ageing and its consequence for the funding of pensions, health and residential care for older people. Finally, and the background of prospective population mobility there is still a need for progress to reduce the barriers to free movement across national boundaries.

The prospects for the further development of social protection in Europe are to be seen in the context of wider debates about macro-economic policy, competitiveness and productivity (Hirsch, 1997). One school of thought holds that the socio–economic model for Europe is one characterised by high labour costs, high productivity and high levels of spending on social security. A contrasting model, derived from both the rhetoric and experience of the United States, is characterised by lower labour costs, lower levels of productivity, lower levels of unem-ployment but also lower levels of social protection. Poverty rates, however, are significantly lower in much of Europe than in the United States. The United Kingdom is located ambiguously between the two models.

Policy-making in the United Kingdom is now more open than it has ever been to ideas and influences from abroad. Membership of the European Union, prospective membership of the European Monetary Union and the imperatives of European employment policy all suggest a future which is shaped by continental traditions, values and policies. But such a conclusion would be premature: if the United Kingdom was ever to become more fully engaged in European debates about the future of social protection their ability to shape policy options along more 'Anglo-Saxon' lines should not be underestimated. The greatest risk is that the possibility of debate, based on sound arguments and robust evidence, is dismissed in favour of insular complacency.

References

Bardone, L. and Degryse, E. (1995) 'Poverty and social protection in the European Union', in ISSA *Social Security Tomorrow: Permanence and Change*, Studies and Research No. 36, Geneva: International Social Security Association.

Bradshaw, J., Ditch, J., Holmes, H. and Whiteford, P. (1993) *Support for Children: A Comparison of Arrangements in 15 Countries*, Department of Social Security, Research Report Series, London: HMSO.

Bolderson, H. and Gains, F. (1993) *Crossing National Frontiers*, Department of Social Security, Research Report No. 23, London: HMSO.

CEC (1992a) Council recommendation 92/442/EEC of 27 July 1992 on the convergence of social protection objectives and policies, OJ L 245 of 26 August 1992.

—— (1998) *Social Protection in Europe 1997*, Brussels: Commission of the European Communities.

Dennett, J., James, E., Room, G. and Watson, P. (1982) *Europe Against Poverty: the European Poverty Programme, 1975–80*, London: Bedford Square Press.

Ditch, J., Barnes, H. and Bradshaw, J. (1996) *A Synthesis of National Family Policies*, Brussels: Commission of the European Communities.

Ditch, J., Bradshaw, J., Clasen, J., Huby, M. and Moodie, M. (1997) *Comparative Social Assistance: Localisation and Discretion*, Aldershot: Ashgate

Eardley, T., Bradshaw, J., Ditch, J., Gough, I. and Whiteford, P. (1996) *Social Assistance in OECD Countries*, Synthesis Report, Department of Social Security Research Report Series, London: HMSO.

European Commission (1996) *Social Protection in Europe*, Luxembourg: Office of Official Publications.

—— (1997) *Modernising and Improving Social Protection in the European Union*.

—— (1998) *Social Protection in Europe 1997*, Brussels: Commission of the European Communities.

Hills, J., Ditch, J. and Glennerster, H. (eds) (1994) *Beveridge and Social Security*, Oxford: Oxford University Press.

Hirsch, D. (1997) *Social Protection and Inclusion: European Challenges for the United Kingdom*, York: Joseph Rowntree Foundation.

Jenkins, S. and O'Higgins, M. (1989) 'Poverty in Europe – estimates for 1975–1985', Poverty Statistics in the European Community, Conference Paper, Noordwijk, Netherlands.

Ploug, N. and Kvist, J. (1997) *Social Security in Europe*, Dordrecht: Kluwer.

Quintin, O. and Chassard, Y. (1992) 'Social protection in the European Community: towards a convergence of policies', *International Social Security Review*, 45(1–2): 91–108.

Robbins, D. *et al.* (1994) *National Policies to Combat Social Exclusion*, Third annual report of the European Observatory to Combat Social Exclusion, Lille: EEIG.

Room, G. (ed.) (1995) *Beyond the Threshold: The Measurement and Analysis of Social Exclusion*, Bristol: Policy Press.

Index